MW00454748

Disclaimer & Copyright

Text Copyright © Siim Land 2016

All rights reserved. No part of this guide may be reproduced in any form without permission in writing from the publisher except in the case of brief quotations embodied in critical articles or reviews.

Legal & Disclaimer

The information contained in this book is not designed to replace or take the place of any form of medicine or professional medical advice. The information in this book has been provided for educational and entertainment purposes only.

The information contained in this book has been compiled from sources deemed reliable, and it is accurate to the best of the Author's knowledge; however, the Author cannot guarantee its accuracy and validity and cannot be held liable for any errors or omissions. Changes are periodically made to this book. You must consult your doctor or get professional medical advice before using any of the suggested remedies, techniques, or information in this book.

Upon using the information contained in this book, you agree to hold harmless the Author from and against any damages, costs, and expenses, including any legal fees potentially resulting from the application of any of the information provided by this guide. This disclaimer applies to any damages or injury caused by the use and application, whether directly or indirectly, of any advice or information presented, whether for breach of contract, tort, negligence, personal injury, criminal intent, or under any other cause of action.

You agree to accept all risks of using the information presented inside this book. You need to consult a professional medical practitioner in order to ensure you are both able and healthy enough to participate in this program. http://siimland.com/

Table of Contents

Introduction

Starve the Animal, Feed the Beast

Imagine yourself in the following situation: You're completely alone in the savannah, you haven't eaten anything for days now, your body bears many scars and it's starting to get dark. In the distance you hear the roars of predators and beasts. You can feel your heart racing, pounding in your chest, and your blood vessels pumping faster than ever before.

Despite all of that, you're not delusional nor very hungry. You wouldn't say *no* to a juicy delicious steak but at the same time it doesn't feel like you're starving. The adrenaline surging through your veins has given you the eyesight of a hawk, the suppleness of a leopard and the strength of a bear. You're simply aware of everything that goes on around you – every scent in the air, every footprint in the dirt, every sound of cracking branches puts makes you more alert. Your mind is sharper than ever before and your muscles are tense, poised for immediate action.

That's exactly what happens when you're in hostile environments and under dreadful circumstances. You don't want to die, and the only way to do so is to become the fittest one around – the apex predator itself.

Such survival scenarios were a part of our aboriginal hunter-gatherer past. Back then, food wasn't abundant and people had to fight for their right to eat every single day. It wasn't a constant struggle, but incredibly exerting nonetheless. Uncertainty was hiding behind every corner and they had to be prepared for anything. They didn't know when or where their meals would come from. Hunters didn't have breakfast lunch and dinner. We tend to take this affluence for granted. Once you go out of food, you'll realize how fortunate its presence actually is.

What's more, hunger is one of the main motivators of our actions. If we want to continue living, then we have to eat. In situations of life and death, our body and mind are willing to do whatever it takes to survive. At those times, we can go further beyond what we thought was possible and expand upon our current limitations. It's sink or swim.

Intermittent fasting is a means of getting in touch with our inner hunter-gatherer. In today's society we're surrounded by food everywhere we go. When you look at the condition the majority of the population is in, then you can see the importance of this abstention. Civilization has brought about its own diseases, which are obesity, diabetes and cancer. The affluence of food has made the average contemporary person overweight, ill, exhausted and slothful.

My name is Siim Land – a holistic health practitioner, a fitness expert and an author. I've been doing some form of intermittent fasting every single day ever since 2012. It's one of the foundational eating strategies I have in my nutritional arsenal. Having perfected this craft, I've managed to improve my health beyond wellness, burn all excess body fat down to single digits, build lean muscle mass very easily, get stronger both physically and mentally, change my relationship with food for the better and make myself more productive. If you follow this protocol, then the same can happen with you.

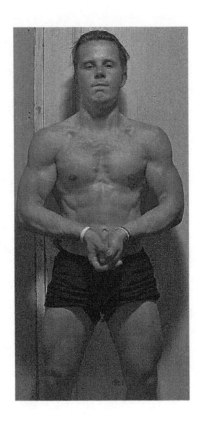

Between these pages lies a much <u>STRONGER, HEALTHIER, SMARTER and HAPPIER</u> version of yourself. Intermittent fasting is extremely effective and easy to do. It doesn't even feel like a diet or anything, because it isn't one. For me, the greatest benefits have nothing to do with body composition, but more with how amazing it makes me feel. It's more of a lifestyle - a way of living that enables you to shed fat and build the physique of an aesthetic Greek god or goddess.

Intermittent fasting is as much a mental practice, as it is an eating protocol. By taming your mind and starving your mindless animal, you'll be able to feed your inner beast and unleash your primal instinct. If you're capable of voluntarily abstain from consuming food, then you're showing very high levels of self-mastery. This will make you better as a human being in everything you do.

In this book I'm going to share with you how to:

- Start intermittent fasting as a sustainable lifestyle.
- Burn all excess body fat down to single digits.
- Build lean muscle mass without putting on fat.
- Never get hungry or feel like you're starving.
- Trigger your lean and mean genes that make you stronger.
- Release the most powerful anabolic hormones within your body.
- Give your hormones steroid-like effects.
- Find your primal instinct and unleash it.

- Eat delicious food and as much of it as you like.

- Feel like Superhuman.

If you're eating something right now, then as Arnold Schwarzenegger would put it: *"PUT THAT COOKIE DOWN! NOW!"*

Let's starve the animal and feed the beast. Let's fast and feast!

Chapter I

The Annals of Intermittent Fasting

The eating patterns of our hunter-gatherer ancestors were highly unpredictable. Quite frankly, they were completely random. Sometimes they had a whole lot – when one of them speared a woolly mammoth, a 10 feet tall beast that weighed about 6 tons. At other times they had absolutely nothing – when there was a drought, famine or wildfires. Whatever the case might have been, they were always in between fasting and feasting. They did both of them intermittently. This cycle wasn't deliberate but created by the scarcity of food in their environment.

Do you know how to catch fish? What mushrooms are safe to eat? When is the best time to collect nuts and seeds? Are you brave and strong enough to hunt mammoths or wrestle with a bear? Probably not.

When you're in an evolutionarily unforgiving environment, then you can't take any chances. Every opportunity you miss can determine your survival. That's why you have to be constantly on your toes and ready to immediately jump into action. For the Paleolithic hunter-gatherer it wasn't a problem to go *from 0 to 100 real quick*, in fact, at an instant. Even in the modern world there are some societies who practice foraging.

An Aborigine hunter has to be willing to exert himself at any given time. I remember a story about a man who killed a huge wild ox at midnight. In the Northern Territory, tribal base camps are quite far away from each other, about 40-70 miles apart. He was 50 miles away from camp and had to run back to call someone for help. Then, he and his brothers dragged the kill back home again. Keep in mind that an average bull weighs at least 1, and they did it in one night. That totaled in around 100 miles of running for the hunter and 50 miles of intense physical labor. He probably did it all while not having eaten anything for at least 16 hours.

The comfortable life of the contemporary world has done us a disservice. As a species we're safer and more fed than ever before in history. We've seemingly overcome the first priority of any organism trying to survive, which is the consumption of calories.

Don't get me wrong, our situation is better than ever before and we shouldn't start chasing wild game for dinner. Instead, it should serve as a reminder of how fortunate we really are and to not take this for granted.

That's why we should all practice some sort of intermittent fasting, daily. Not only is it good for our health but also is a way to express our gratitude. It's one of the best eating habits to have.

An important notion is to distinguish fasting from starvation. One is *voluntary* and *deliberate,* the other is *involuntary* and *forced upon.* It's like the difference between suicide and dying of old age. Abstention from food is the art of manipulating our metabolic system and can be done for many reasons. Malpractice might look like the person is starving, but if done correctly it's very healthy and good for you.

Our body can only be in 2 metabolic states

- Fasted – meaning that there are no exogenous calories consumed at all.

- Fed – there is some food circulating the blood stream.

Even consuming small amounts of food will put you into a fed state. It doesn't matter whether you eat 200 calories or 1000, you'll still be shifted out of a fasted state.

That's why I intermittent fasting is a lot better than caloric restriction. If you're feeding yourself, but in inadequate amounts, then your body will most definitely perceive it as scarcity. You'll be causing more damage than good. If you do it the wrong way, you'll end up like someone from the concentration camps.

Daily caloric restriction decreases metabolism, so it's easy to presume that this would be magnified as food intake drops to zero. However, this is wrong. Once your food intake stops completely (you start to fast), the body shifts into using stored fat for fuel. The hormonal adaptations of fasting will not occur by only lowering your caloric intake. In the case of being fasted, your physiology is under completely different conditions, which is unachievable by regular eating.

Starvation happens when there is not enough nutrition to be found *e.g.* when you go on a weight loss diet and restrict calories. While fasting, the organism is almost never deprived of essential nutrients, unless you lose all of your body fat. These fuel sources are mobilized from internal resources.

Fasting isn't a mechanism of starvation because your metabolism will be altered. This shift won't occur entirely if you continue consuming food, even when you've reduced your calories to a bare minimum. It's actually a lot healthier way of losing weight, as you'll be burning only fat, not muscle. When on a restrictive diet you'll never make the leap and to keep your energy demands at a balance you begin to cannibalize your own tissue. When in a fasted state, this can be circumvented.

Some Fast Fasting History

Fasting is one of the most ancient healing practices in the world. Hippocrates, the father of modern medicine, said: *"To*

17

eat when you are sick, is to feed your illness". He recommended abstinence from food or drink for almost all of his patients.

Plutarch said: *"Instead of using medicine, rather, fast day."* When an animal gets sick or injured, its immediate natural instinct is to stop eating. You've probably felt something similar, when you get a fever. Once the crisis is over, and you've healed, the appetite will return back to normal.

Before Hippocrates, the infamous god Hermes Trismegistus, or Thoth the Atlantean in Egypt, said to have invented the art of healing. He used fasting to unveil the secrets of the cosmos by cleaning his body and purifying his mind.

In Ancient Greece, consuming food during illness was thought to be unnecessary and even detrimental, since it would stop the natural recovery process. There was also a widespread belief, that excessive food intake could increase the risk of demonic forces entering the body. Perhaps obesity and slothfulness so many are plagued by today?

The Greeks believed that abstention from food improved cognitive abilities as well. Pythagoras systematically fasted for 40 days, believing that it increases mental perception and creativity. He also wouldn't allow any of his students to enter his classes unless they had fasted before. So did Plato, Socrates and Aristotle – all of the great philosophers. They frequently abstained from food intake for several days.

This would seem reasonably effective, as the only way for a hunter-gatherer to end their starvation was to get smarter and more efficient at catching game. Toolkit complexity is linked with increased hunting and fishing practices[i], as traps and toggle-headed harpoons require more intelligence to make than simple digging sticks. Unlike plants, animals run away from us and if you want to eat them, you have to come up with better ways of catching them. This ever-imposed stress on hunting societies was probably one of the major driving forces behind the development of our species.

Intermittent fasting is also practiced by most of the religions of the world. Christianity, Judaism, Buddhism and Islam all instruct abstention from food in some shape or form. Similar teachings are preached in philosophical, moral and tribal codes. It's commonly thought of as a definite way of creating a communion between God or other divine deities.

In Jainism, following prescribed rules of fasting and practicing certain types of meditation leads to transcendent states that enable the person to dissociate themselves from the world. It's described as an out-of-body experience, a completely altered state of consciousness.

The Islamic holiday Ramadan forbids the Muslim from eating during the day when the sun is out. They go through a short period of 12-16 hours of fasting for spiritual as well as medicinal purposes. It also restricts the consumption of water, making the people dehydrated and their experience that much more lucid.

In the Quran it's said: *"Fasting is prescribed for you as it was prescribed for the people before you so that you may become pious." (2: 183) The purpose of fasting is to illuminate the heart and mind of man aimed at bringing about comprehensive revolution in his individual and collective life."*

The Ramadan is one of the most studied types of fasting. It's proven to have great health benefits, such as an increase in red and white blood cells, reduction of inflammation, body fat etc.[ii]. However, all of the advantages of this practice aren't very clear, because the Muslim tend to gorge themselves at night and before sunrise. So, there's both fasting and feasting.

Christianity, especially Roman Catholicism and Eastern Orthodoxy, advocate a 40-day fast before Easter, during Lent, and before Christmas, during Advent. Since the Second Vatican Council (1962-1965), this has been modified to allow greater individual choice, with mandatory fasting only on Ash Wednesday and Good Friday. There are also periods where certain food types are restricted, such as meat.

The Mediterranean Diet is considered to be one of the healthiest ways of eating in the world. It's famous for comprising of a lot of fish, salad, olive oil, nuts etc. People who live at the shores of the Mediterranean Sea have less heart disease, diabetes and live longer. The American researchers quickly made the conclusion that it has to do with the large amounts of mono-unsaturated fats and lack of meat and butter.

But that's not necessarily the reason for their improved health. What they didn't notice was that the Greek Orthodox Church also advocates a lot of fasting. In fact, an average religious Greek fasts more than 200 days a year. That's probably the hidden secret to their longevity.

The only religion that prohibits fasting is Zoroastrianism, because of its belief that such asceticism will not aid in strengthening the faithful in their battle against the sources of evil. But intermittent fasting has extremely empowering effects, which actually make the practitioner stronger, healthier and smarter. Those traits are definitely useful for battling anything. I'm going to share with you the ways of doing so in the coming chapters.

Buddhist monks are said to be able to fast for up to 72 days. While in deep meditation, they lose their desire for anything and experience a blissful state of mind. I myself have felt something similar but not to the point of spiritual enlightenment or religious revelation, unlike the Yogis of India or Native Americans. Maybe I haven't just fasted long enough.

When your body is deprived of food you begin to see things differently. Of course you'll be thinking about eating, but this focus can be redirected to other things. Once you master your emotions concerning the situation you get a feeling of relaxation and calmness.

Abstinence from food is required in preparation for many rituals in cultures across the globe. In Greece it was thought of as a must for getting into contact with supernatural forces. In the Hellenistic mystery religions, such as the healing cult of Asclepius, the gods were said to reveal their divine knowledge in dreams and visions only after the devotee had been fasting for an extended period of time.

Aboriginal witchdoctors and healers would probably also attest to this, as it's said to cause ecstatic epiphanies. In some Native American tribes, fasting is practiced before and during a vision quest. Among the Evenk of Siberia, shamans got their supernatural powers not from a divine revelation or journey, but after an unexpected illness. After the initial dream they fasted and trained themselves to see further visions and control spirits.

The Sumerian epic hero Gilgamesh sought to find immortality to revive his fallen companion Enkindu. He travelled the landscape for months and walked through the darkest of caves until he reached a sage. During his entire journey he hadn't eaten anything – day and night - and was thus considered enlightened and worthy of receiving a small potion from the Fountain of Eternal Youth. It didn't help him though, because it got stolen by a serpent while the man was sleeping. He reached immortality nonetheless, as his people kept telling his story and carried his achievement through centuries.

Moses received the Ten Commandments on Mount Sinai after having fasted for 40 days and 40 nights. In the Old Testament fasting would prepare a prophet for divine revelations (Daniel 10:2-14).

Siddhartha by Herman Hesse is a story about Gautama Buddha that talks about his life and path towards enlightenment. In the book, he is a monk and a beggar that comes to a city and falls in love with a famous seductress Kamala. He makes his move on her but she asks: *"What do you have?"* One of the well-known merchant does so as well: *"What can you give that you have learned?"* Siddhartha answers the same way in both cases, which leads him to ultimately getting everything he wants. He said: *"I can think. I can wait. I can fast."*

- I can think: You possess good judgement and you're able to make good decisions.
- I can wait: You have the patience and perseverance to play for the long-game without misallocating your resources.
- I can fast: You are capable of withstanding difficulties and challenges. Fasting trains you to control your physiology and makes your mind more resilient.

These three traits are extremely useful for living life according to your own terms. This book will teach you how to cultivate all of them.

However, it's not the fasting *per se,* that enabled Buddha to reach enlightenment. At first, he would fast for many days so that he could be liberated from desire. As the story goes, he ate only a grain of rice and a sesame seed per day. His muscles waned and he got so thin that he could touch his spine by pressing on his stomach. He lost his strength to meditate and realized the wrongness of his ways. Then a young herds maid offered him some milk porridge, which he gladly accepted. His strength was reinvigorated and he understood Buddhahood. By stopping fasting, and eating just enough, he practiced moderation instead. That's what this book is about – periodically abstaining from food and then compensating for the lack with adequate amounts of nutrition.

Fasting has been used as a means of protest as well. Mahatma Gandhi fasted at least 14 times, 3 of which lasted for 21 days. His non-violent stance against the British Empire finally granted India freedom. The longest political fast was done for 74 days by Terence MacSwiney after his arrest during the English-Irish unrest in 1920[iii]. Unfortunately, he died because of that. On that same day, Joseph Murphy, another member of the Irish Volunteers, also died, after having been on a hunger strike for 76 days. To this date, the hunger strike has been used as a weapon of political persuasion in Ireland, with 10 members of the Irish Republican Army having fasted to their deaths in prison after 45 to 61 days[iv]. Goes to show how seriously people take this, especially the Irish. Luckily, this book isn't as extreme as these examples, to say the least.

For health, fasting has been advocated by many, even since the Middle Ages. Luigi di Cornaro was a Venetian aristocrat living at 15th and 16th century. By the age of 40 he had accumulated severe illnesses thanks to excessive eating and drinking. No medication or physician was able to help him and his days seemed to have been numbered. However, there was one doctor who, contrary to popular practice, suggested periodic strict abstinence from food. Cornaro survived and rid himself from all his diseases. When he was 83 years old, he wrote his first treatise *Tratatto de la Vita Sobria (A Treatise of Temperate Living)* and died at the age of 102. Talk about a comeback!

During that same era, the Swiss-German doctor Paracelsus was also in favor of this: *"Fasting is the greatest remedy, the physician within."* In the medical community he's famous for revolutionizing the medical sciences, by utilizing empirical observations from nature, rather than referring to ancient texts. He also gave zinc its name, calling it *zincum* and noted that some diseases are rooted in psychological conditions. For all of his patients, he advised intermittent fasting. Not something you see in today's doctors who would much rather prescribe drugs.

In the mid-1800's, E.H. Dewey, MD, published a book called *The True Science of Living*, in which he said: *""every disease that afflicts mankind develops from more or less habitual eating in excess of the supply of gastric juices."* Basically, consuming too much food too often, without letting the body repair itself. It's like shoving more and more trash into a garbage bin until it starts to overflow. Why not simply take it out?

Since the 20th century, as doctors became more knowledgeable about the human body, fasting became increasingly popular as disease treatment and prevention. Some methods lasted more than a month, allowing only the consumption of water, non-caloric beverages, exercise and enemas. Other modified fasts allowed the intake of about 200 to 500 calories a day, which came from vegetable soup, broth, honey or milk.

There have been many non-obese persons who have recorded their prolonged bouts of abstention from food. Alexander Jacques fasted for 30 days in 1887 and for 40 the year after[vvi]. An Italian *professional faster*, Signor Succi, said that he had done at least 32 fasts of 20 days or more, with his longest ones lasting for 40-45 days[vii].

For obesity, fasting has been used as effective therapy for a long time. Overweight patients have been put on fasting regimens of up to 159, 200 and 249 days[viii]. The longest recorded fast lasted for 382 days (1 year and almost 1 month). It was done by a 27-year old obese man, who lost 125 kg (276 lb) in the process[ix]. After that much time, did he even know how food tasted like? Imagine that first bite...

However, the average person in the Western world hardly experiences the sensation of hunger nor do they enter a fasted state. This is a shame as it will not only prevent them from getting all of the benefits but also make them more fragile and dependent of their illusory food.

Chapter II

The Physiology of Fasting

Intermittent fasting (IF) is a way of eating (or not eating), where the food consumed is restricted to a certain time frame. This means that no calories whatsoever get put into our body in any shape or form. In a way it's simply timing when you eat. There are several patterns to this, all of which we will go through shortly.

The two governing states of metabolism are fed and fasted. The former is when we're using the macronutrients eaten, that have been digested and are now circulating the blood stream. The latter happens when all of that fuel has run out and our gas tank is empty, so to say. It happens after several hours (7-8) of not eating.

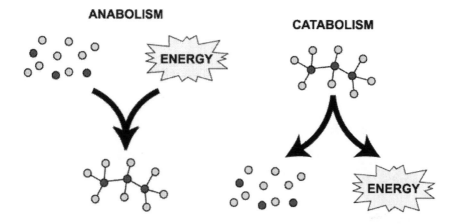

They're the different sides of the same coin. There are only two options: (1) eating and storing calories, (2) not eating and burning calories. Caloric restriction will still keep you in a fed state, a malnourished one, but still. Think of them as the Ying and Yang of metabolism.

You might think that no machine cannot operate without any fuel. That's true only for mechanical things, but us humans are organic and a whole *nother* being. Even though there is no fuel readily available we're still able to function. In fact, to excel at it.

In a fasted state there are several ways to produce energy.

The body's default fuel source is glucose, which exogenously (externally) comes in the form of sugar and carbohydrates and is stored endogenously (internally) as glycogen. The liver can deposit only 100-150 grams and our muscles about 300-500 grams. They're used for back-up.

Liver glycogen stores will be depleted already within the first 18 to 24 hours of not eating, almost overnight. This decreases blood sugar and insulin levels significantly, as there are no exogenous nutrients to be found.

Insulin is a hormone released by the pancreas in response to rising blood sugar, which happens after the consumption of food. Its role is to unlock the receptors in our cells to shuttle the incoming nutrients into our muscles, or when they're full into our adipose tissue (body fat).

HOW DOES INSULIN WORK?

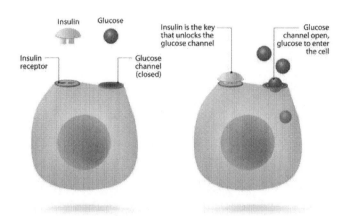

The counterpart to insulin is glucagon and also gets produced by the pancreas. It gets released when the concentration of glucose in the blood stream gets too low. The liver then starts to convert stored glycogen into glucose. This initial phase of fasting is characterized by a high rate of gluconeogenesis (the creation of new glucose) with the use of amino acids from bones and muscles.

As fasting continues, the liver starts to produce ketone bodies which are derived from our own fat cells. Lipolysis (breakdown of stored triglycerides in the adipose tissue) and ketogenesis increase significantly due to fatty acid mobilization and oxidation.

Ketosis can occur already after 2-3 days of fasting. Triglycerides are broken down into glycerol, which is used for gluconeogenesis, and three fatty acid chains. Fatty acids can be used for energy by most of the tissue in the body, but not the brain. They need to be converted into ketone bodies first.

The degree of efficiency depends on the individual and how adapted they are to ketosis. It's a topic for a whole *nother* book (which I have already written – check out my other work in the end of this one) but simply put, it's a metabolic state in which fat is the primary fuel source, instead of glucose, and can be achieved either through fasting or by following a ketogenic diet.

Fasting induces ketosis very rapidly and puts the body into its more efficient metabolic state. The more keto-adapted you become the more ketones you'll successfully utilize. At first, the brain and muscles are quite glucose dependent. But eventually they start to prefer fat for fuel.

After several days of fasting, approximately 75% of the energy used by the brain is provided by ketones. This also allows other species, such as king penguins to survive for 5 months without any food[x]. Protein catabolism decreases significantly, as fat stores are mobilized and the use of ketones increases. Muscle glycogen gets used even less and the majority of our energy demands will be derived from the adipose tissue. This can be accomplished by following a well-formulated ketogenic diet as well, which actually mimics the physiology of fasting almost entirely.

Keto adaptation cannot occur in the presence of excess carbohydrates. Ketones are actually a third fuel source. The Krebs cycle is a sequence of reactions taking place in our mitochondria that generate energy during aerobic respiration (a fancy way of saying breathing normally). When glucose enters this metabolic furnace it goes through glycolysis, which creates the molecule pyruvate. In the case of fatty acids, the outcome is a ketone body called acetoacetate, which then gets converted further into beta-hydroxybutyrate and acetone. Ketone bodies may rise up to 70-fold during prolonged fasting[xi].

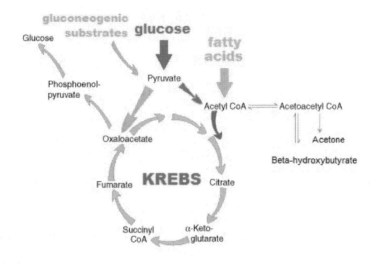

The difference between pyruvate and ketone bodies is that the latter can create 25% more energy. On top of that, the by-products of glycolysis are advanced glycation end-products (AGEs), which promote inflammation and oxidative stress[xii][xiii], by binding a protein or lipid molecule with sugar. They speed up aging[xiv], and can cause diabetes.

Fasting also skyrockets human growth hormone exponentially within the first few days to maintain lean body mass and muscle tissue. Afterwards it does so less significantly because protein catabolism gets reduced to almost non-existent levels.

In this state, the majority of the body's energy demands will be met by the use of free fatty acids and ketones.

Why Fast

Now that we know what it is you might ask, why should we do it? Why abstain from eating voluntarily when it's readily available? That's a natural response.

Our species has followed the eating pattern of feast and famine ever since its genesis. Even today, hunter-gatherer societies have to fight for their food every single day and they sometimes can't make ends meet. They won't die because of that but instead simply get hungry from time to time.

In nature, food isn't as abundant as in our contemporary world of supermarkets. To be honest, it's an illusion, making us blind to how fortunate and unorthodox it actually is. Not only can we eat but also have a variety of products to choose from, too many, to be honest.

It's quite paradoxical that the majority of people in the world go to bed while starving every single night, but at the same time almost everyone in the Western society is obsessively obese.

The Pareto principle applies here perfectly. He was an Italian economist and in his 1896 paper showed that, in most cases, about 80% of the effects come from 20% of the causes. 80% of the wealth belongs to 20% of the people, 80% of car accidents happen to 20% of the drivers, 80% of the food is consumed and stored as fat in 20% of the world's population etc. Mainly it's used in economics, but this 80-20 rule, or the law of the vital few, is evident in the distribution of calories and obesity as well.

Our civilization has reached a point where we don't have to worry about our most primary needs as much and can now spend more time on other activities that develop us further as a species. There's nothing wrong with that. In a perfect world no animal would have to kill another one and everyone would always be fed and satisfied. However, we don't live in such a place yet, at least for the time being.

Nevertheless, despite the fact that we're surrounded by calories of all sort we still should do intermittent fasting. If you look at the rise in obesity and cardiovascular disease this abundance has bestowed us with then you definitely would realize the necessity of it for some people. However, these are only the obvious self-evident reasons. There are even more benefits to it which will improve the health and well-being of the lean individuals as well.

Chapter III

The Effects of Fasting

Fasting completely alters the physiological conditions of our body. Most of it has to do with shifting into ketosis, which is achievable with a low carb diet as well. However, there are also other adaptations specifically characteristic to a fasted state.

The effects of fasting are very broad and cover both physical, mental and spiritual benefits. Once we stop eating for a while, our perspective on life changes and so does our body.

There are many beneficial and even empowering adaptations that occur during the abstinence from food. The most profound ones have to do with health, but they can also translate over to other domains as well.

Cellular Repair

Fasting is like a miracle cure, as many philosophers and physicians of the past would agree. The Renaissance doctor Paracelsus called it the *"physician within."* Because it triggers the body's own healing mechanisms it can be effectively used as treatment for almost any disease.

This is caused by the principle of _autolysis,_ which is an organisms ability to selectively self-digest and remove unwanted material within the body, without touching vital structures.

When in a fasted state the body actually conducts a lot of the necessary repair mechanisms. It detoxifies the organism by triggering a metabolic pathway called _autophagy_, which removes waste material from cells[xv]. In the process, inflammation throughout the body and overall oxidative stress get reduced[xvi]. This fights all illnesses.

Disease is not a natural state to be in. The body is smart enough to fight it. We simply have to get out of our own way and let the automatic mechanisms set in to do their job. Constant eating directs all of our energy into digestion and doesn't create time for housekeeping. Because of the crap most people are eating, waste starts to accumulate and their body becomes a garbage bin. To prevent cancer and increase lifespan[xvii] we need to intermittently abstain from eating and recover[xviii].

Increased Fat Oxidation

Fasting is also the healthiest and easiest way to reverse obesity. We already know about how bad caloric restriction is for us. There's a big difference between losing weight and burning fat. You probably know on which side you want to be.

Before you can burn fat, you have to first "release" the fatty acids into your blood stream through a process called lipolysis. Then they get transported to the mitochondria where they'll be oxidized into energy.

During rest, our muscles start to use more fatty acids for fuel. When fat burning increases so does the amount of Uncoupling Protein-3 in our muscles. As little as 15-hours of fasting enhances the gene expression for UP-3 by 5-fold[xix]. We'll be using ketones to feed our lean tissue more effectively.

In a fasted state we begin to use our own body fat as fuel. This not only promotes body composition but also teaches us to produce energy despite the lack of calories. As a result, we experience less hunger and fatigue by not being dependent of food in order to feel great. It's an important and vital thing for our survival which we don't want to lose.

By being constantly fed we're never really converting fatty acids into the blood stream and are simply burning the food we've digested. This will definitely slow down weight loss, if not put a harsh halt to it completely. In the case of an unexpected famine we would be dumbstruck for a while because our body doesn't have enough reference experience. In a nutshell – fasting allows your body to take a break from storing fat, and start burning it.

Hastened Metabolism

Contrary to popular belief, intermittent fasting doesn't slow down the metabolism but actually increases it by 3.6% after the first 48 hours[xx]. Even further, 4 days in, resting energy expenditure increases up to 14%.

Instead of slowing down the metabolism, the body revs it up and puts it into higher gear. This is probably caused by increased adrenaline so that we would have more energy to go out into the savannah and find some food. The scarcer calories become the more detrimental it is to succeed in hunting.

People think that if they skip breakfast the body will hold onto its own body fat and store every calorie in the next meal. Think about it. Does your body really think it's starving after not eating for a day or is it simply your primal mind playing tricks on you? Like said, the pattern of feast and famine is something our species is adapted to. It's just that people have lost these pathways of fat oxidation and think they're dying when they don't eat 6 meals a day. Their metabolism simply needs to be made more resilient.

Increased Insulin Sensitivity

In a fasted state, we actually become more efficient with the food we eat, instead of storing it all. With the lack of calories, especially carbohydrates, we become more insulin sensitivity[xxi], meaning that we need less of it to lower our blood sugar levels back to normal. In the case of resistance, the pancreas can't pump out enough to get the job done which leads to hypertension and disease. Fasting can actually reverse insulin resistance and reduces overall blood sugar levels.

Lowering insulin gets rid of excess salt and water in the body, which is caused by carbohydrates in the first place. Insulin is the key hormone in the regulation of our metabolism and the main driver of obesity and diabetes. Fasting and a low carb diet are great ways of controlling its expression.

There's no reason to be concerned about malnutrition during fasting, because our fat stores can deposit almost an infinite amount of calories. The main issue is rather micronutrient deficiencies. Potassium levels may drop slightly, but even 2 months of fasting don't decrease it below a safe margin. Magnesium, calcium and phosphorus remain stable because 99% of them are stored in our bones. The man who fasted for 382 days maintained such a lengthy period with no harmful effects on health thanks to taking a simple multivitamin. That's all you need to survive for that long.

Boosts Human Growth Hormone

Another anabolic mechanism that gets increased is human growth hormone (HGH). After 14-18 hours of fasting it does so by 1300-2000%[xxii]. It not only promotes tissue repair, body composition and metabolism but also preserves youthfulness. The hormone of eternal life and youth – the Holy Grail of longevity.

Growth hormone plays a key role in the metabolism of all macronutrients. Its normal secretion fluctuates throughout the day and increases significantly during the first hours of sleep at about 11-12 PM.

After 3 days of fasting, HGH increases dramatically in non-obese individuals, but flats out after day 10[xxiiixxiv]. In obese people, there is little to no reported rise after fasting from 14 to 38 days [xxv]. Hypothetically, this happens as a response to preserving lean tissue. I would suggest that beyond that point the body simply becomes extremely well keto adapted and reduces both the overall energy demands as well as increases the efficient use of ketones as fuel.

What goes hand in hand with HGH is insulin-like growth factor (IGF-1). It's one of the major growth factors in mammals, which together with insulin, is associated with accelerated aging and cancer. Just 5 days of fasting can decrease it by 60% and a 5-fold increase one of its principal IGF-1-inhibiting proteins: IGFBP1[xxvi].

By the same token, it's an all-encompassing anabolic hormone, like insulin, that makes everything within the body grow – the good (muscle), the bad (fat cells) and the ugly (tumors). It gets reduced during fasting but also gets stimulated by it, as with physical training.

Additionally, testosterone increases as well. During my 48-hour fasts I usually experience higher libido than normally. Even though there's no direct reason for it, I have a feeling of risen masculinity and T-levels. It's not aggressive energy, but more like my determination heightens and my focus narrows down completely.

Intermittent fasting creates the perfect environment for anabolism not catabolism as a lot of people think. Being constantly fed results in the over-expression of insulin and IGF-1, which is not optimal. You want to activate them in very specific conditions. Occasional fasting is a great way to control and use them only when you want to.

You don't have to take the steroids to release these anabolic hormones. They're already a part of our physiology. We simply have to turn on some of our genetic switches and become fat burning beasts.

Longevity and Life-Span

Fasting induces oxidative stress because of producing a surge in free radicals, the molecules mostly associated with aging. This further stimulates a gene called SIRT3[xxvii] to increase the production of *sirtuins*, which are protective proteins of longevity. In mice they extend lifespan. There are no studies on humans, but it probably has similar effects.

The rise in free radicals is actually beneficial, by triggering protective pathways. If the body is intermittently exposed to low levels of oxidative stress, it can build a better response and cope with it better.

On top of that, autophagy and insulin sensitivity keep the body clean and healthy. Too much junk will damage our mitochondria – the power plants of our cells. Ketosis actually increases our mitochondrial density, giving us more energy, and so does intermittent fasting. The combination of those two can help us live a lot longer.

Having combined both of these strategies I definitely feel like I've put a halt to my aging process almost entirely, at least slowed it down significantly. I'm still 22 and I shouldn't show any signs of getting older in the first place, but based on my gut feeling I'm expecting to live past 100.

My insulin is almost never elevated and my blood is clean of free radicals. After ditching the carb, eating a lot of healthy fats and doing intermittent fasting, my skin has never been clearer and my nails are perfect.

Rejuvenescence

By the same token, fasting has a characteristic that's perfectly natural to life. It's the ability of living things to regain youthfulness. This physiological term is called *rejuvenescence.*

Experimental scientists have demonstrated this on lower forms of life. They deprive some creatures back from adulthood to their embryonic stage of life, as if they were reborn. This has been done several times, meaning that the animal has reached an old age and then has been reverted back to its youth, over and over again.

For humans this probably won't work, but man can definitely benefit from the same physiological characteristics. At the University of Chicago, Carlson and Kunde fasted a 40-year old male for two weeks and discovered that his cellular physiology was that of a 17-year old. This happens by ridding the cells of toxic metabolic accumulates.

One of the features of youthfulness is seen in the cell to nucleus ratio. Youthful cells have a preponderance of nuclear material, while old and senile cells have a dominance of cellular material. Autophagy keeps the cells refreshed and circulates between old and new building blocks.

Fasting will also rejuvenate your psychological youthfulness. You get a breath of fresh air and can give your brain some reasons to enhance its functioning. Frequent eating also dulls the mind and makes you mentally more slothful. The hungry hunter's cognition was as sharp as a knife.

Cancer and Tumors

There are some good reasons to consider fasting as something that could potentially cure cancer. One of the first studies in this field showed that it not only prolonged life but reduced the prevalence of breast cancer tumors in rats[xxviii]. Another one done on mice found out that 48-hour fasting effectively protected normal cells but not cancer cells against high doses of chemotherapy and also alleviated its side-effects.

The reason might be that there's simply not enough food for cancer cells to feed upon. While fasting, blood glucose levels drop and ketone concentration increases. The #1 fuel for tumors is sugar and they commit cellular suicide through starvation. It probably isn't enough to cure the disease completely in humans, but it's a step in the right direction.

For healthy people, intermittent fasting can instead be used as disease prevention. Increased insulin sensitivity and *autophagy* are quite good predictors of longevity. It's the most natural antioxidant there is. It heals, repairs and regenerates the body. These qualities are greatly enhanced during a fast and can cure diseases that don't go away while eating.

Bolstered Brain Power

While intermittent fasting we will experience mental clarity. It also increases levels of a hormone called brain-derived neurotrophic factor (BDNF)[xxix], a deficiency of which has been implicated in depression and various other similar problems.

New brain neurons get formulated, which is a process called *neurogenesis* Intermittent fasting makes one mentally sharp and reduces brain fog. It sharpens cognition, increases learning memory and enhances synaptic plasticity[xxx], improves our stress tolerance[xxxi] and protects against neurodegenerative disease[xxxii]. Ketosis may increase seizure thresholds in epileptic patients as well, which is stimulated by fasting.

Evolutionarily it promoted ingenuity – to find new ways to getting food etc. When faced with famine, the only way to survive was to get smarter.

Fasting can be used as a way to boost your mental powers. Artists and writers in the past usually abstain from eating during their most creative circuits. Michelangelo painted the ceiling of the Sistine Chapel vigorously day and night, rarely coming down to eat or even sleep.

Franz Kafka's short story *The Hunger Artist* is about a man who is a professional faster. He travels across the towns of Europe and puts himself on display in a cage. The hunger artist earns his living by fasting for 40 days. Unfortunately, the people don't share his idea of self-restraint and think that he's cheating in some way. They assign butchers to guard him at night, to ensure he doesn't eat anything. What's even more humiliating is that these men deliberately turn a blind eye to him, as if to allow him to steal some food. The hunger artist sings to prove his credulity but no one believes him.

He fasts for 40 days at once and then changes location. Even though he could go longer than that and actually wants to do it, his business partner forbids him because the spectators lose their interest. Eventually, professional fasting goes into total decline because of the audience wanting more exciting forms of entertainment. The hunger artist then joins the circus and gets put in a cage next to ferocious lions. At this point, deliberate abstention from food resembles an art form itself, but it's also a humiliating spectacle. I'm going to cut the story short for now and will return to it again later.

Back to the effects of fasting...

After the body has shifted from using glucose to burning fat for fuel, appetite gets reduced dramatically. This is because the brain gets abundant energy from ketones. You'll be able to direct your psychic energy onto other more demanding activities.

What follows is a sense of well-being and euphoria. The explanation might be that the accumulation of acetoacetic acid produces a mild intoxication similar to that of ethanol[xxxiii]. You'll be literally high on keto.

Potential Side-Effects

There may also be some negative consequences to fasting. Headaches, dizziness, lightheadedness, fatigue, low blood pressure and abnormal heart rhythms are all short-term. Some people may experience impaired motor control or forgetfulness.

But these are all symptoms of withdrawal, not fasting. Because most people rarely get to use their own body fat for fuel, they become too dependent of glucose. It's like an addiction that makes them crave more sugar.

When I first started practicing intermittent fasting I experienced some hypoglycemia (low blood sugar response) but nothing serious. I simply got a bit lightheaded whenever I stood up too fast. After going on a ketogenic diet those signs have disappeared completely.

Any mental hindrance is caused by an inner energy crisis. Once the body adapts to utilizing fat for fuel, the brain will accept ketones and will also reduce hunger.

Fasting may cause some flare-ups of certain medical conditions, such as gout, gallstones or other diseases. This is yet again not because of the physiological effect of fasting but because of the overall high amounts of toxins in the body. The adipose tissue is more than a caloric pantry. It also stores poisons and infections that we digest. The food we eat is the most immediate point of contact we have with the world around us. Unlike the skin, our gut is the one who does all of the absorbing. Once you start breaking down triglycerides, those same venoms will be released into your blood stream again and need to get flushed out. There may also be some nervous stomach, irritable bowel of diarrhea. That's why fasting is an effective detox tool, as it cleanses the organism completely.

In comparison to all of the empowering health benefits of fasting, these few side-effects are minute and not guaranteed. They may or may not happen. What's certain is that they will be alleviated after time.

Why then have we been lead to believe that fasting is bad for us? Medical doctors and supplement companies all preach the consumption of 6 small meals a day. Why? I'm not going to be pointing any fingers or calling anyone out, but simply put: <u>there's no money to be made from healthy people.</u> How do you prescribe a pill of fasting that's completely free?

Fasting is perfectly natural and incredibly powerful tool for many purposes. The most obvious ones have to do with body composition and fat reduction. For someone like me who is already as lean as I can be, the best benefits have to do with using ketones as fuel and increased longevity. It's one of the staples in my nutritional arsenal and something we should all be doing, no matter our condition.

Chapter IV

Deliberate Abstention of Food - The Power to Choose

Based on the physiological and psychological benefits of being in a fasted, it would be stupid not to practice IF. However, the greatest good lies beyond that.

For me, voluntarily abstaining from food is about more than restricting my eating window. It's a great way to control one's caloric intake but first and foremost it's about controlling oneself.

Intermittent fasting is a display of self-mastery and strength of willpower. Most people don't even have control over their own mind and therefore gorge themselves constantly.

Why is this so anyway? Why do people eat food past satiety until indulgence and obesity?

The reason for that has to do with our primal origins again. You see, the change in our environment from scarcity to abundance has happened too quickly. We may live in the modern world, but our body thinks it's still in the ancestral landscape.

Because of this *"evolutionary time-lag"*, our brain is always trying to motivate us to consume the most valuable sources of calories – salt, sugar and fat. They're with the highest nutrient density and can be easily stored for the dark times to come. Unfortunately, those times are happening less and less.

The deadly combination of salt, sugar and fat is like a drug, as it stimulates our taste buds in an addictive way and lights up the reward mechanisms in our brain. Michael Moss' book titled the same way talks about how fast food companies have deciphered this secret code that makes us crave more food. It's called the bliss point – the specific amount of those 3 ingredients, which optimizes palatability. There's not too much nor too little, but just enough. By themselves, they're not inherently bad but when together they cause conflicting metabolic and hormonal effects within the body that leads to diabetes and obesity.

The reason why some people can't get enough enjoyment from healthy food is that their bliss point is too high. Refined carbohydrates, sweets, pastries and pizzas have overstimulated their taste buds. They simply can't even feel the taste of anything less than that. To keep up with their primal urges they want to increase their sensations even further. Instead of being satisfied, they keep craving for more and more.

With self-mastery you can circumvent that and "hack" your bliss point. If you habituate yourself with less stimulating food that has real natural flavor you're teaching your brain to enjoy it more. Your taste buds will light up even when consuming something bland because they're sensitive and haven't been burnt out.

Intermittent fasting adds to that, as it acts as a sugar detox, by resetting your taste buds. It makes you remember how good healthy food actually tastes like. They say ignorance is bliss...Wait until they take their first bite after a 24-hour fast

What Makes Us Human

Eating is as much a neurological as it is physiological process. The human brain consists of the following:

- The basal ganglia, also called the reptilian brain is the most primitive part of our brain. It governs balance, territoriality, mating, feeding and other instinctual activities.

- Then we have the center part that comprises the „limbic system", which consists of the septum, amygdalae, hypothalamus, hippocampal complex, and cingulate cortex. This the mammalian or monkey brain – the brain of emotions and social hierarchies.

- Finally, at the front, there's the human brain, the cerebral cortex. This is where rational thinking is, especially at the pre-frontal cortex. It's the most recent step in the evolution of the mammalian brain and gives the ability for language, abstraction, planning and perception.

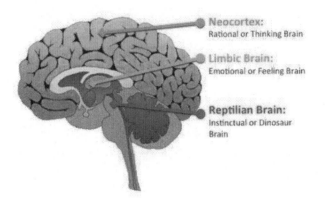

Neocortex:
Rational or Thinking Brain

Limbic Brain:
Emotional or Feeling Brain

Reptilian Brain:
Instinctual or Dinosaur Brain

If you wonder where you are, then the answer is: right behind your forehead, in the prefrontal cortex. That's where the idea of the „SELF" gets created. But it's more than that. As you can see, there is even some correspondence in here with eating as well.

- The reptilian brain governs your physiological processes, such as the need for food and shelter. It's concerned only about the body.
- The Limbic system is based on emotion, feelings and thoughts. It's the mind.
- The neocortex is above the other two because of being capable of rationality. It's the crown jewel of evolution and human development. I can't tell you whether or not

that's exactly where your soul lies, but it's still higher above than the other two.

If you think that food is scarce and you should consume every single calorie in sight, just in case, then you're behaving under the influence of your reptilian brain. It's the first stage of development in mammalian brains. This will lead to insulin resistance and diabetes.

Another thing that causes binge eating is leptin resistance. It's the *satiety hormone*, that regulates the feeling of hunger. Leptin's role is to signal the brain that there's dire need for calories. Once we get full it sends another message, saying that we've had enough. However, if we're resistant to it then the lines of communication will be cut short and our mind will never get the information that we've received enough food. In this case, the body is satisfied but the brain is still starving and keeps on craving for more stuff.

Leptin resistance is caused most by emotional binge eating. It's governed by the Limbic system, that influences the way we feel and what social relationships we follow. It usually goes hand in hand with insulin resistance, as it is created by the consumption of simple carbohydrates and sugar with a lot of fat at the same time. This is the most common cause of obesity and diabetes.

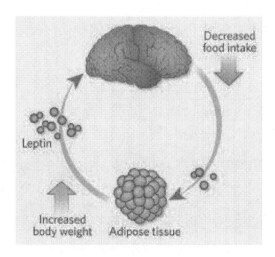

Self-mastery, on the other hand, is about being more conscious as a person and aware of what creates these urges and how to overcome them. It comes from the pre-frontal neocortex – the crown jewel of our current evolution. This human brain is characterized by rationality, the ability to see oneself in space, time and in relation with others. The heightened level of consciousness is caused by being able to understand the consequences of one's actions and to see them enroll in the future.

Our behavior is constantly governed by these 3 brains. Which one dominates most depends on how strong your pre-frontal cortex is. In essence, how human you are. If you act on higher levels of consciousness, you're aware of the presence of your reptilian instinct and its emotional sidekick. You still need to satisfy your physiological needs, but thanks to self-mastery you can deliberately do so in moderation.

In nature, scavengers gorge themselves as well. Whenever they catch a prey, they eat as much as possible. For animals like the hyena and wild dogs, food is scarce and they never know where their next meal is going to come from. The reason why they're still lean and fit is that they simply aren't surrounded by that many calories. They're obese in their mind but their body is just under very demanding conditions.

A predator, on the other hand, only eats when its hungry. A lion stops eating and leaves once it has reached satiety. When that happens the scavengers, like hyenas and vultures, fly in to get their share. The lion knows that it's the apex predator of the savannah and can always catch his dinner whenever it feels like it. When it's full and satiated, it can sit under a tree with a zebra right next to it and not care.

Even more, the wolf will bury a carcass underneath the ground and returns to it later. It won't eat when there's danger around and is willing to endure some more hunger. The scavenger will eat whatever they can find and whenever. They do it on the run and are concerned only about eating.

The predator thinks of food as abundance, whereas the scavenger sees it as scarcity. Granted, they're different animals, but I think you get my point.

Obesity is caused by acting like a zombie. People eat like scavengers because they can't control their primal urges. They don't realize that they're actually being mind-controlled by their selfish genes and hormones. It's almost not their fault. They've simply fallen into a downward spiral of mindless slumber.

But the lion doesn't voluntarily fast. It still follows the feeling of hunger and is driven by the desire to eat.

Herein lies the point that distinguishes us from the rest of the animal kingdom. Our meta-cognition enables us to rise above this evolutionary circuit and see ourselves from an outsider's perspective. We're aware of the presence of these primal urges, well at least some of us, and can CHOOSE to take control of them.

Scavengers eat whatever fits their mouth and the lion follows the growling of its stomach, but deliberate intermittent fasting is a way to make our own terms with our physiological development and to take the reins of evolution into our own hands.

What's even greater about this is that it can reset the body's physiological and psychological condition. Once we abstain from food, the body can start to heal itself. This will also reverse leptin and insulin resistance, as our taste buds will be shortly liberated from the stimulating effect of processed junk.

It's the miracle cure within, that cleanses and purifies the mind as well.

It changes our relationship with food, which is probably the most important notion here. Not only will we become more grateful for a meal but will also realize how fortunate we really are. Every bite gets that much more enjoyable, if we haven't eaten for a while.

It's natural and not something we have to fear. It's evident that it doesn't harm but actually empowers us. Being able to go without food for an extended period of time while not suffering any consequences is an amazing ability to have. If we know that we're not actually starving, then our confidence improves and we can attain self-mastery by rising above these initial reactions and urges.

Chapter V

The Enslaving Effect of Food

Don't get me wrong. I'm a total foodie and love to eat. It's just that I like to do it on my own terms and less frequently.

Constant feeding is enslaving. The reason why big herbivores, like elephants and cows, eat all of the time is that they need to meet their daily energy requirements that would support their large size. Plant foods don't have a lot of calories and therefore they have to dedicate most of their waking hours to chewing and digesting food. Talk about a sad unfulfilling life.

Breaking down food and digesting it requires a lot of energy. Energy, which is the first priority for any organism, and which takes away resources from the brain.

Us humans have managed to develop such large neocortices thanks to eating more nutrient dense foods, such as fatty meat. Once our body was satisfied, our cognition had the opportunity to flourish and consciousness to reach such high levels.

Also, the anthropologist Dunbar and Aiello have found that there's a significant correlation between relative neocortex size, group size and social grooming in non-human primates[xxxiv]. This forced our early ancestors to develop language, which wouldn't have happened, if our brains had stayed small.

We wouldn't have created civilization and started creating art if we had to spend the majority of our time thinking about food. That's why I love the ketogenic diet. In combination with intermittent fasting, it removes any feeling of hunger or cravings.

Instead of feeling obligated to eat several meals a day, we should realize that intermittent fasting does us more good than harm and it actually improves the quality of our life.

During antiquity, the rich folk of Rome and Athens would not eat almost anything during the day and were occupied with other things. At night they would feast like kings and relax. As a child I remember reading about their grandiose dinner parties from history books. People would have all types of incredible dishes – meat, fish, wild game, fruit, olives, bread, cheese, wine etc. Looking at sculptures and paintings, you can't say that they were fat. Quite the opposite. Most Greeks had a Herculean physique and were not only ripped but also jacked. How did they manage to pull it off? Intermittent fasting.

Instead of eating during the day, they would feed their slaves instead. Yes, the household servants had constant access to food in the pantry and kitchen. They weren't starving but were being deliberately fed.

Why did the rich feed their slaves? So that they wouldn't get in touch with their primal instincts that gets stimulated by abstinence from food. Their minds remained dull and bodies weary because of being in a constantly fed state. So it happens with caged animals. The lion in a zoo and the lion in the savannah are completely different. One is a sleeping *pussy-cat* – slothful, domesticated, waiting for its next meal. The other one is a raging beast – strong, fast, sharp and a king of its realm. Fasting releases adrenaline and increases fat oxidation, that give us more energy and puts us into hunting mode. It wakes up the predator within.

How to Break Free

Let's return to the physiology of fasting for a moment.

As you can remember, the 2 governing metabolic states are fed (anabolism) and fasted (catabolism). Eating stimulates the parasympathetic nervous system, which is the "rest and digest" or "feed and breed" mode. It's meant to make us more calm and relaxed but at the same time slothful.

Ever wonder why you get that post-lunch dip? It's because your body wants to digest food and makes it a priority. The majority of your energy gets allocated to the breakdown and absorption of nutrients. You want to curl up and go to sleep, so that you could store that energy.

On the flip side, fasting stimulates the sympathetic nervous system – the "fight or flight" response. The purpose here is to make us more alert by releasing adrenaline and giving us more energy. It's meant to assist us in either catching prey or running away from predators.

Have you ever felt how going hungry sharpens all of your senses? You become more sensitive to the scent and sight of food. Abstinence narrows down your focus and increases your concentration. By default, the reptilian brain makes you search for calories, but if you control the urge with your neocortex, you can direct that heightened attention to anything else.

The catabolic nature of fasting actually stimulates anabolism. Initially it causes damage, which then sets the stage for supercompensation and enhanced cellular growth. It's the same with resistance training – during the workout you're making your muscles weaker which then get stronger during rest.

While fasting, we're causing physiological stress to the body, which conditions our entire organism to handle it better in the future. Without there being a necessity for it, nothing would grow. If we're mostly in a safe environment, we'll soon let our guard down. That's why we should deliberately trigger these responses so that we could maintain our expertise and deadly finesse.

Catabolism stimulates anabolism and *vice versa*. To build new tissue we need to first break the old one down. A shaky foundation won't support any solid structure for long. Hormonal stimulation through intermittent fasting flips the switch in between.

Absence of food and starvation is a signal that makes the body want to maximize food utilization and protein synthesis, making us more efficient with our fuel and causing certain adaptations to occur.

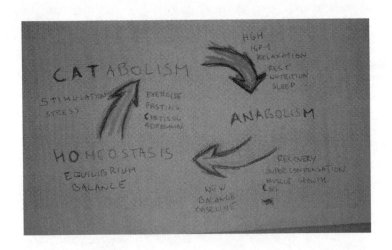

<u>**This phenomenon is called *HORMESIS*.**</u>

In biology, when you expose an organism to only a very small dose of a lethal or damaging stimuli, such as physical training, cold exposure, heat, sunlight, fermented foods and yes – intermittent fasting, you will get a beneficial response.

The body will always try to maintain a stable core temperature, blood sugar levels and caloric balance. Hormesis disrupts homeostasis, the state of inner equilibrium. Intermittent fasting creates an environment, which requires certain adaptations to take place, so that we could survive. As a result, the organism will then adapt to these new conditions and gets stronger.

But the key notion lies in how much stimulus you're creating. If it's too much for the organism to handle, then it will actually get weaker. What makes a poison deadly is the dosage. That's why after catabolism there needs to be anabolism and fasting has to be coupled with feasting.

Strategic periods of undereating, followed by overeating will make the body react in a positive way. By adapting to the stress intermittent fasting creates, we will become stronger, healthier and better at burning fat for fuel. It raises the ceiling and power of our homeostasis. Our habitual mode of being will be that much greater.

So it was in Ancient Rome. The rich were sharper with their mind and had more mental toughness. The poor were stuck in a vicious cycle of constant feeding, which prevented them from ever mustering enough courage or energy to rise above. It was the result of falling into a downward spiral of slavery. Until Nero, there wasn't a single emperor who was obese, but he was also insane.

Of course, there were other factors that determined this, but this was one of the main reasons. The poor were larger in numbers and could've easily overthrown their masters. The issue wasn't that they didn't have the ability or strength to do so. It's just that their inner beast had been tamed and domesticated by a seemingly innocent force.

One of the major uprisings against the Roman Republic was led by a gladiator called Spartacus. He was born and raised in the wild steppes of Thrace and was only brought into the arena later in his adolescence. Unlike the other slaves, he hadn't been beaten into servitude. Spartacus probably didn't do intermittent fasting but still managed to summon enough courage and determination to take action. The taste of freedom was still fresh in his mind and he couldn't just let himself be dominated. His cause wasn't successful and he was killed in battle but it's better to fight for one's rights and die rather than to live like a slave.

Seneca, one of the most famous Roman Stoic philosophers, would deliberately practice abstinence from not only food but from all other earthly possessions. He was the richest banker in the city but still would live like a beggar at least one day of the month. For him it was a way of conditioning himself to not be dependent of his abundance and increase his gratitude for what he had. He said: *"Set aside a certain number of days, during which you shall be content with the scantiest and cheapest fare, with coarse and rough dress, saying to yourself the while: "Is this the condition that I feared."*

There's something so admirable about such behavior. It shows that you approach life with open hands and abundance. The scavenger mindset has been completely set aside and there's no scarcity in one's behavior. It also shows bravery and courage of heart. Doing the uncomfortable and getting comfortable in doing so.

Intermittent fasting liberates us. It frees our mind from having to eat so often while at the same time causes a lot of empowering physiological adaptations in the body. The stress response that gets created makes us stronger, better, faster and quicker in our minds. It keeps us alert and on our toes.

In our current environment we don't need extreme survival skills and metabolic efficiencies but they're still invaluable parts of our biology. Ketosis and autophagy don't happen in of themselves but are triggered by the inner conditions of the body. In the presence of elevated insulin and blood glucose levels, fat oxidation and ketone utilization get put to a halt. We don't want to lose touch with our inner beast and primal instinct. We might need it again in the future.

Chapter VI

Choose Your Weapon of Fasting

If by now you've realized that there are immense benefits to intermittent fasting, you probably want to know when to do it? To be honest, there isn't a definite answer to be given here. Everyone has different lives and time schedules.

Actually, it doesn't even matter when, as long as you simply do it. The length of the fast isn't as important either. After a certain amount of time we'll have reaped all of the benefits and can stop fasting, without going through several days.

Here are a few ways of doing it.

- **24-hour fast.** This is the most basic way. It doesn't even have to mean that you actually go through a day without eating. Simply have dinner in the evening, fast throughout the next day and eat dinner again. This one is also prescribed by the author of *Eat Stop Eat* Brad Pilon. The frequency depends on the person but once or twice a week should be the golden standard. An active person who trains hard should do it less often than a sedentary person. Some people also go longer than that but I don't see any reasons to do so. Going without eating for more than 2 days just doesn't accomplish as much as we already get from that 24 hours.

- **16/8 time frame every day.** This is my favorite strategy, popularized by Martin Berkhan, which I'm doing daily. You fast for 16 hours and have a feeding window of 8. Simply skip breakfast and have it during lunch instead. By that time all of the HGH and other hormonal benefits will have reached their peak. It's also the time where our body has managed to digest and remove all of the food and waste from the previous day. In my opinion, we should all be following this. It's an optimal way of eating by consuming food only when it's necessary. We don't even have to be as strict with it. Instead of following 16/8 we can do 14/10, 18/6, 20/4 or whatever fits the situation. The point is to simply reduce the amount of time we spend in a fed state and to be fasting for the majority of the day.

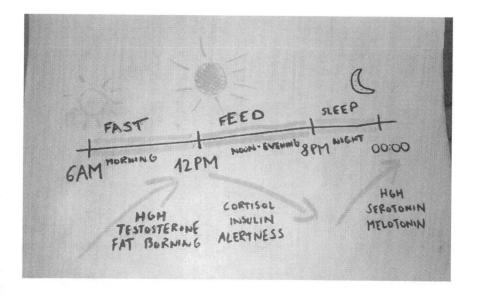

- **The Warrior Diet** is a fasting protocol created by Ori Hofmekler. The entire concept is based around ancient warrior nations, such as the Spartans and Romans, who would be physically active throughout the day and only eat at night. At daylight they would only get a few bites here and there and would consume a lot of calories in the evening. This diet follows the 20/4 timeframe with one massive meal eaten at dinner.

- **Fasting for several days**. Although very effective for weight loss, I don't see immense benefits in doing this for healthy individuals. Autophagy and detoxification will certainly increase but I would like to think that similar results will be achieved with daily intermittent fasting, such as the 16/8 window. The frequency might actually be a lot better than the intensity. However, doing a fast for several days at least once a year sounds like a wise idea, as it will completely detoxify the body and will also clear metal toxicity.

- **Breakfast and dinner.** As a final resort you can follow the pattern of 50-50, meaning you have breakfast early in the morning, go through the day without eating and have dinner. This way you'll fast for about 8-10 hours and actually do it twice in one 24-hour period. It's not ideal but still better than 6 meals a day. At least you'll be able to not become too dependent of the food and can get the most of the benefits.

There are also approaches like *The 5:2 Diet* and *Alternate Day Fasting*, which include fasting but allow the consumption of about 500 calories on days of abstention. I wouldn't recommend this, because caloric restriction won't allow all of the physiological benefits of fasting to kick in. You want to shock the body and go straight to zero for the greatest effects.

Another thing to consider is protein fasting. In a nutshell, you occasionally reduce your daily protein intake dramatically, almost to a zero. It's a great tool to reduce inflammation, kick-start weight loss and to protect yourself against tumors, cancer and aging.

By doing protein fasting once a week, you're allowing your body to induce *autophagy*. You'll be self-digesting your own tissue. It might seem like you're cannibalizing yourself and starving, but in reality *autophagy* is required to maintain lean body mass and it actually inhibits the breakdown of muscle in adults[xxxv].

It also improves mitochondrial functioning, resulting in better sleep. *Autophagy* is required for healthy brain cell mitochondria[xxxvi]. Regular fasting does the trick as well, but regularly limiting your protein intake is another great way to do this. This makes your cells find every possible way to recycle proteins endogenously. At the same time, they bind and excrete toxins that are hidden in your cell's cytoplasm[xxxvii].

Being chronically protein deficient is horrible for the brain and body. The trick is to do it intermittently, like with fasting. After skipping protein intake completely (24-hour fast) or reducing your intake close to zero (about 15 grams), you'll supercompensate for that scarcity and increase its utilization.

This makes sense from the perspective of evolution as well, because hunters didn't have slabs of stakes lying around like we see in the supermarket. A woolly mammoth was killed only every once in a while and when that happened it was a feast.

How Long Should I Fast

Fasting is good for you but we should still consider other lifestyle factors. The most important variables are frequency and your current level of leanness. If you decide to fast every day, then you don't need to go longer than 16 hours. Choosing to do it once or twice a week means that you should scale up the intensity and go for the entire 24-hours.

It might seem that the longer the fast – up to 36 hours – the greater the health and disease-prevention benefits. However, that's a double-edged sword. Lean muscle mass is a critical component of longevity, healthy living and being ultimately fit. Longer fasting doesn't cause as much muscle catabolism as you'd think, but it definitely won't enable you to build or maintain it for long. It will also negatively affect nutrient intake. You won't be able to get in your essential micronutrients – minerals, vitamins and phytochemicals – which may lead to deficiencies.

The leaner and more physically active you are, the less you need to fast. First of all, there's not much benefit to gain from that frequent abstinence. You'll hit a point of diminishing returns quite quickly after which there are no great advantages. Secondly, if you want to workout and keep making progress, then you simply won't be able to do so as much. Fasting is powerful but good quality nutrition is still the foundation of getting stronger.

This book doesn't advocate for extreme types of fasting that exceed the 3-day mark. It's definitely a great detox and we should fast for at least 48-hours several times a year. If you choose to do any such experiment, then do so at your own risk. Instead, I'm more of a proponent of eating less frequently and practicing some IF intermittently every day. Being healthy overall is a much more sustainable strategy and a well-formulated whole foods diet already protects you from a lot of disease and other ailments.

But it's important to ask yourself: *"why do I want to fast?"* If you're doing it for weight-loss then you should also re-consider your other lifestyle factors, such as diet and training. It's not a quick-fix. *Oh, I'll just eat whatever junk I can find and then fast for a week...* Unless you have over 200 pounds to lose, you don't have to take it to such extremes. Trying to break the 382-day world record doesn't sound like a good idea either.

You can choose your weapon of fasting depending on the situation you're in. If you don't have access to good food or simply feel like skipping a meal, then do the 20 hour fast. At other times you can do less. While travelling it's so easy to do this. You don't want to consume a lot of processed food anyway and IF helps to avoid that.

Chances are, if you're used to eating 4-6 meals a day you may find transitioning over to intermittent fasting difficult. Having less frequent meals forces your body to adapt and may take some time until your ketogenic pathways get reinvigorated. You can "ease into it," by starting to eat less often at first and then shortening your feeding window even further.

For me, changing my eating schedule happened quickly. First I started off with the 16/8 approach and pushed my breakfast until 10AM. Dinner was at 6PM and because of that I tended to go to bed hungry. This didn't work for long and I kept pushing my first meal later into the day. It was a lot more sustainable and satisfying, as I got to eat more food and sleep satiated. You have to find out what works for you. It's all one big scientific experimentation, in which the subject of the study is you (n=1).

The best advice I can give you is to simply start. Jump in head first and expect nothing but the best results. You can ease into it and start with skipping breakfast at first, but in my opinion, it's a lot better to simply shock yourself completely. This will wake your metabolism up and tells the liver that it's time to start using fat for fuel. That's what I did. I read about IF and after a couple of days started practicing it. I've never looked back again. The same happened with my first 24- and 48-hour fast. I had always wanted to do it, but had never gotten around to do so. One day I was having dinner and thought to myself: *"what the hell, might as well get it over with."*

The key is to practice IF daily, in some shape or form. You don't want your feeding window to oversize the time you spend fasted. 12-12 isn't ideal either. It's better to always be on the negative side of things, if you get my point. This way your body has to always guess whether or not it will get some calories and will have to utilize more fat for fuel.

These eating strategies are all a lot better than the standard 4-6 small meals a day recommendation. Which leads me to a very controversial topic that needs to be clarified...

Chapter VII

The Breakfast Myth

"It's the most important meal of the day! Wake up, eat a lot of fruit and cereal to kickstart your metabolism and give yourself energy!" You've probably heard this from nutritionists and fitness gurus countless times. To be honest, I'm quite sick of it.

Actually, they're right. Breakfast is indeed the most important meal of the day, as it determines our metabolic state for the rest of the day, as well as the next. However, it doesn't mean we should be having it.

Eating first thing in the morning doesn't have any beneficial effects. After an overnight fast we're in an advantageous state of increased fat oxidation. Our liver glycogen stores have been depleted and we're in mild ketosis.

Within a few hours, other hormonal activities will speed up and we'll empower our body. Growth hormone gets released and our insulin sensitivity improves. Also, testosterone increases and our cells go through the repair mechanisms of autophagy. The reason is that the body is in a semi-catabolic state and will become more efficient with nutrient partitioning and shifts into a higher gear of fat burning.

Having breakfast with a lot of sugary cereal, fruit, or a whole grain bagel will put a harsh stop to all of these adaptations. Tony the Tiger is wrong. It's not grrrreat! Causing an insulin response at any other time of the day can prevent fat burning completely or at least slow it down significantly. Another reason why you would want to eat a ketogenic diet.

The stress hormone cortisol is also the highest. It rises at about 6-8 AM so that we could become more alert for the coming day. This increases our adrenaline and fat oxidation even further. Why not take advantage of this short boost? It would be a shame to pass out on all of these adaptations. The stage is set, we just have to get out of our own way.

When you go to bed at night, you release the most growth hormone. Having fasted in the morning, you condition your body to do it more than 1300-2000%[xxxviii]. If you ate, then you won't be doing it nearly as much.

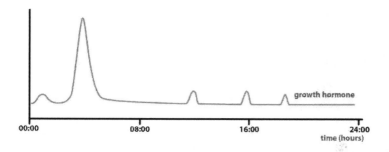

There is also a circadian rhythm to hunger (day and night cycles), with a ditch at 8AM and a peak at 8PM[xxxix]. A study found that despite the extended overnight fast, paradoxically, people aren't as ravenous in the morning and they tend to not want much breakfast. You'd think that the longer they've spent fasting the hungrier they'd get, but the opposite happened. No matter how long their fast had lasted, the participants still reported less desire to eat after waking up. Instead, the internal clock increased appetite in the evening, independent of food intake and other factors. This makes perfect sense, as after an overnight fast we're in mild ketosis and utilizing fat for fuel. It also means that no matter how much whole grain cereal you stuff down your throat once you open your eyes, you'll still get hungry by the evening. The difference is that you'll have skipped all of the hormonal adaptations and have already consumed a lot of calories during the day.

This I've noticed in my own hunger signaling as well. In the morning I don't have a lot of desire to eat immediately. Only after taking the first mouthful does the desire arise. Before that I'm actually very satisfied and don't even notice any difference. It probably has to do with the fact that we've been conditioned by our society to start feeding right away. The work horse has to be just nourished enough to do its job. If it gets too strong and powerful though it may become a problem...

Why is it thought that you would gain weight if you eat in the evening? It's probably based on past experiences. But that knowledge has nothing to do with meal timing. Instead, people gain weight when they have big dinners because they've already spent the majority of the day feasting. Having breakfast, lunch and multiple snacks in between will have already made them consume a lot of calories. Now, they've already reached their caloric maintenance and can easily go over to a surplus. They simply don't have a nutritional plan and are winging it.

On the flip side, those warriors and aristocrats in Ancient Rome did the opposite – they were underfed and thus had a lot of calories to consume. Some of it was involuntary, as soldiers didn't have many opportunities to eat, other than in the evening. The rich, however, did it deliberately and were perfectly fine.

Another warrior race were the Huns and Mongolians. Attila the Hun was called the *Scourge of God* by Romans, because he terrorized both the Western and Eastern Roman Empire with his pillaging.

Genghis Khan lead the Golden Horde and created the largest empire the world has ever seen before, spreading from the shores of China to the gates of Vienna. It covered India, Middle-East, Asia Minor and Central Asia. They're also the only nation in history who has successfully conquered Russia.

Nomadic people are also constantly on the move. They ride and hunt the majority of the day and don't have that much time to eat. The steppes created a different type of character, which the Romans found hard to fight against.

A Mongolian rider would put a piece of meat under his saddle in the morning and tenderize it by the evening. Instead of eating something on the run like a scavenger, they patiently waited for the occasion, in which food reached its greatest value. They managed to thrive in battle because they were intermittently fasting and in deep ketosis.

That's why I would always recommend not having breakfast. Actually, we can never really skip it as the first thing we put into our mouths, despite the time, will shift our metabolism from being fasted into a fed state. We're simply having it later in the day and still getting our nutrients.

Why Am I Hungry?

Hunger is created by the hormone called ghrelin, that is produced by the gut to stimulate appetite. It signals the brain that the body is running low on fuel and it is time to eat something.

However, it doesn't necessarily mean that there is an energy crisis. It's more like a pre-cautionary message that lets us know when we have reached the lower ends of our storage. Think of it like the gas light of your car.

The biggest reason why us humans have to eat so many calories is to feed our hungry brain. It's the most expensive tissue we have. Making up less than 5% of our body weight, it demands about 20% of our total energy expenditure.

Leptin resistance and the release of ghrelin happen because of the brain perceiving energy as scarcity. These hormones ought to motivate us to consume more food, even when there's no immediate necessity for it. We'll happily store any excess into our adipose tissue.

However, the brain shouldn't require a lot of calories to maintain its functioning. Once our immediate access to energy within the body has run out we still have a lot of stored fuel with us. From the perspective of evolution, we shouldn't experience hunger because of facing exhaustion. The energy stored in our adipose tissue would keep us alive but we still get hungry. Looking at how large our fuel tank really is, it seems that the issue isn't how many calories we have but how effectively we use them.

If you think that you have to eat first thing in the morning, then riddle me this: *"Why do you think you need to have breakfast?"*

The reason can't be to prevent yourself from starving to death. Nor can it be to *"kickstart your metabolism"* or prevent gaining fat. When you look at my body composition, which is at single digits year-round, and how much I train, which is every day, then the reason can't have anything to do with some sort of an advantageous metabolic state.

My body is constantly under very demanding conditions, yet I do not suffer any negative effects of undereating. I'm incredibly lean, muscular, strong and fit – all while not having breakfast. Please, tell me more that you need to stop your muscles from cannibalizing themselves and prevent yourself from getting fat.

Warriors were also constantly underfed during the day. A Roman legionnaire had to carry all of his belongings with him during military campaigns. They would have to march for hours, with at least 40 lb of equipment on their backs. Of course they ate something here and there, but they definitely didn't have pre-, intra- and post-workout shakes with them. Unless some extra terrestrial gods, the Anunnaki or the like, bestowed them with some sweet whey protein powder.

The reason why you think that you may break down your own muscle is that your body doesn't know how to use its own stored fuel. Our adipose tissue can deposit almost an infinite amount of energy. Even the leanest of individuals with less than 5% body fat carry around more than 20 000 calories with them at all times. What about those who are overweight then.

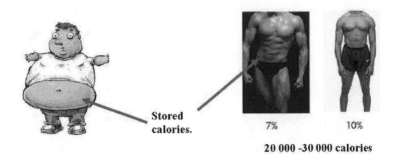

Stored
calories.

7%   10%

20 000 -30 000 calories

Experiments of prolonged fasting on obese people show that they get hungry once their adipose tissue gets depleted and they reach lower amounts of body fat. This happens in conjunction with increased Neuropeptide Y. In the Bible, Jesus was said to have fasted for 40 days and 40 nights, before he got hungry.

You get hungry because you can't access that infinite supply source. This is the result of contemporary eating habits, such as snacking and having 6 small meals a day. Frequent eating will never lead to complete satiety. Even when you have one big meal at lunch, you will still continue to crave food because you're used to having it very often. Remember, the body adapts to exactly the conditions it gets exposed to.

What Causes Sugar Cravings

The same thing applies to sugar cravings. Every time we consume something sweet, the reward endorphins in our brain light up. We release a lot of the "feel-good" chemicals, such as dopamine and serotonin.

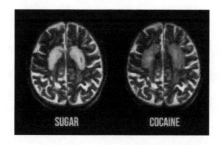

As you can see, the brain's reward system lights up the same way on sugar as it does on hard drugs. In neurological terms, binge eating and drug addiction are the same thing[xl].

This happens so that we would be motivated to repeat our actions in the future. Our taste buds are designed to recognize sweetness and fire up every single time. Feeling good after eating something sugary puts us on a short high and makes us want more.

At the same time, that quick burst of energy will meet its quick downfall. After eating carbohydrates, our blood sugar levels rise. In response, the pancreas releases insulin to lower it back to normal. As a result, we will experience a drop, because insulin is clearing our blood stream from glucose and shuttling it into either muscle or fat cells.

This sharp high is followed by a steep low that causes mild hypoglycemia. A drop in blood sugar levels makes us feel sleepy and drowsy instead of energized.

Now the body is facing an energy crisis. The brain will then scream out for more energy. Because the best fuel source it can think of is glucose, it will create sugar cravings.

The reasons for sugar cravings is to make the body search for easily storable energy and to prevent hypoglycemia.

However, both of them are not justifiable in most situations. If a person has a lot of body fat, then they are carrying around stored energy with them at all times. Yet they can't seem to lose sugar cravings at night. Any other time of the day, really.

Sugar cravings are an effective evolutionarily stable strategy, but only in environments where finding energy is difficult. Calories in the modern world are more than abundant.

You shouldn't have sugar cravings or feel hungry after a meal at all because of just having consumed calories. If you do, then you might have some blood sugar problems.

To get rid of sugar cravings and reduce the feeling of hunger, we have to teach our body to burn fat instead. Becoming fat adapted means that we know how to use fat for fuel very efficiently. As a result, we will have access to almost an infinite amount of calories stored in our adipose tissue.

Intermittent fasting is a great strategy for reversing leptin resistance and reducing the expression of ghrelin. If you want to completely free yourself from sugar addiction, then **you need to reset your body's taste buds.**

Following a short period of ketogenic eating acts like a sugar detox. You'll clear your liver and muscle cells from excess glucose and begin to use fat as fuel. This will truly liberate your mind as well from wanting carbohydrates and makes your body independent of sugar.

Your bliss point gets lowered, but your happiness will increase. Imagine how good you'll feel once you get out of the rut of craving more and more stimulation without ever reaching satisfaction. Ridding yourself from the desire is where the solution lies. Go straight to the root problem, which is inefficient energy usage, and don't simply alleviate the symptoms.

These metabolic pathways don't happen in of themselves and need to be tapped into. You have to teach your body how to burn fat and a period of adaptation is necessary. That's why you should do the ketogenic diet at least once, as it will reset your body and reinvigorates your fat burning mechanisms.

It's true that your basal metabolic rate will slightly decrease with less frequent eating. But that's not necessarily a bad thing nor will it equal fat gain. You begin to need fewer calories not because your body is starving but because your metabolism gets more effective. Occasional intermittent fasting will initially speed up the process by 3-14%. A kickstart is needed only when there's a necessity for it. Small meals will allow your body to become slothful, whereas it's better to be sharp and poised for immediate action. With enough conditioning you'll be able to plug into the largest fuel tank of them all.

The desire to have breakfast is therefore not caused by physiological necessity but by psychological hunger.

These two things are distinct from one another. They also include the notions of self-mastery and higher levels of consciousness.

Physiological Hunger	Psychological Hunger
• Empty feeling in the stomach	• You are not physiologically hungry
• Stomach pangs	• If you wait, the hunger goes away
• Light headedness	• Is emotionally triggered through sight, smell, or habit
• Headache or irritability	

Most people eat simply out of boredom. They have nothing else to do other than to walk between the fridge and the couch. This is sad and should be addressed immediately. Snacking is already one of the worst habits to have. It has nothing to do with needing energy. If you feel like it, then you should practice intermittent fasting. This goes straight to the underlying issue, which is your body's inability to use its own fat for fuel.

Are you afraid of hunger? This almost phobic fear of going hungry is completely irrational. Our society is already teaching us that we should eat frequently and an empty stomach is a dangerous sign of starvation. In reality, it activates our primal instinct and puts us into hunger mode, in which we're more alert, stronger and sharper. Fasting makes us *hungrier for life.* If you're controlled by it and give in too easily, then you're being enslaved by your urges, just like the servants in Rome.

First, you should realize that it's not going to harm you. It's mainly a brief sensation that occurs according to your habitual eating schedule. Your body is simply asking you, whether or not you still remember that previously it has received food at this exact moment. If you skip this urge, then you're conditioning yourself to not be influenced by it.

Fasting allows you to re-conceptualize hunger. Instead of linking it with panic, lethargy and desire[xli], it can be associated with success, self-mastery, pride, or simply ignored. You'll actually become more mindful of your urges and realize that most of the time you're following your habitual eating patterns.

Excruciating hunger with pain involved is a different story. It probably won't happen during fasting, but only when your body is chronically depleted of essential nutrients. Self-mastery is about controlling not torturing yourself. You should listen to your urges and understand them correctly. Learn how to differentiate between physiological hunger and psychological cravings.

Be More Mindful, Be More Human

I despise mindless eating on the run as well. Simply putting something into your mouth doesn't mean that your mind actually realizes that you've fed. The scavenger is the one who has to take an advantage of every opportunity of eating in sight. It can't realize that food doesn't equal scarcity and that skipping a meal isn't bad. The predator knows that going hungry will only strengthen it and won't gorge itself.

Imagine yourself being obese and watching TV. Next to you is a bag of chips, which you're constantly digging into. One handful after another you keep on shoveling that food into your throat without even noticing it. At one point you reach the bottom and open up another bag – the vicious cycle continues. As sad as it seems, there are too many people like this. They already have leptin resistance and it's only a matter of time until diabetes and other cardiovascular diseases catch up with them.

I would much rather make every meal special and savor it. Rather than eating mindlessly, we should bring our complete attention to the dish. Follow along with me on this short fantasy mind trip. Smell the aroma of your favorite food. Is it steaming hot, or something cold? Allow your taste buds to already light up before you even take a bite. The juices are flowing in your mouth and you look at the plate in front of you. It's a beautiful sight, especially if you're breaking your fast. You're already anticipating your first mouthful but don't get too attached to it. Let your motive be in the act itself, not the reward.

As Leonardo da Vinci said: *"The average person looks without seeing, listens without hearing, touches without feeling, eats without tasting, moves without physical awareness, inhales without awareness of odour or fragrance, and talks without thinking."* In addition to mindless eating, we're being less mindful in all areas of our life. People don't know how to control their emotions because of having distanced themselves from their physiology. Fasting re-creates this intimate relationship we all should have with our body.

Mindfulness is about being aware of oneself in the present. It's recognizing what goes on in our immediate surroundings and being capable of creating modules of ourselves in the future to come. In so doing, you're raising your level of consciousness, which is the creation of your higher self, the pre-frontal cortex and even beyond that.

As you're reading these lines, are you completely present? Can you truly say that you're entirely HERE and in the NOW.

Take a notice of what goes on around you. What are the sounds you hear in your ears, the smells you smell with your nose like? Bring your total attention to the soles of your feet, your breath and be aware.

More importantly, what goes on inside you? What sort of feelings and sensations are you having? Are you being controlled by your moods, or have you managed to achieve self-mastery and rise above them?

Rather than falling victim to our ego and getting high-jacked by our emotions, we have to opportunity to take control of them. Mindfulness enables us to always behave from the perspective of our higher self. It's what makes us human.

Eat your food and be grateful for it. Feel how the flavors enroll in your mouth – salty, sour, tenderness, not too much and not too little. Before going for another mouthful, enjoy the moment and let the current stimulus to pass (it takes about 10-15 seconds). You don't have to do this in slow motion, as it might look like in your head. Eat at normal speed, but at the same time be completely mindful of the process.

For me, skipping breakfast is incredibly enjoyable and easy. During my morning hours I get the most of my creative work done. In fact, it's 9AM as I'm writing this book. My mind is extra sharp and I'm able to formulate top notch literature, *sans food*. Leonardo himself practiced fasting and he was a genius.

Think how much more productive we can be by eating less often. Food is like a civilization's obsession. Don't get me wrong again. I love eating as well as cooking. On top of being a writer I also consider myself an up to par chef. It's almost therapeutic and a special occasion. But it's just that – a significant event that picks up its value only because of its low frequency. If I were to do it 3 times a day I wouldn't enjoy it nearly as much.

With intermittent fasting you don't have to think about meal prepping either. I've never been one of those guys who cooks all of their meals of the week and packs them into Tupperware. Who would want to eat that? Of course you can heat it up but when you're on the run you would have to consume it cold. That's not very tasty. A scavenger eats carcasses that have been left to rot. The predator eats a fresh kill with the blood being still warm.

I have chickens – 10 of them. They're great pets to have because of their ability to lay eggs. In my opinion, eggs are the #1 source of protein in the world, especially if they're pastured and come from homegrown animals. They're full of essential fatty acids, omega-3s, DHA, EPA and cholesterol, all of which are detrimental for cellular growth, repair, cognition and the production of hormones.

Every morning I open the hatch and let them outside of the barn. Every single time they roar out, as if something is chasing them. They immediately start eating food that I've laid there. The rest of the day they're simply picking bugs, cackling and behaving like any other birds. I'm not advocating that my chickens should do fasting, because I want the eggs. It's just that every time I see how ravenously they eat I can't forget about how controlled they are by their reptilian brain. Their following the desire to eat that gets signaled by their unconscious urges. The *neocortical* decision of choosing to rise above that circuit becomes that much more appealing.

Ultimately, you have to come to terms with what relationship you want to have with food. Do you eat to live or live to eat? Intermittent fasting can improve your health, body composition and eating habits. At the same time, it enables you to still enjoy delicious meals. Actually, the quality and taste of them gets better. As the saying goes: *"You never know what a good meal tastes like, until you haven't had it for a long time."*

Chapter VIII

Controlled Randomness

It's only recently in the evolution of our species that food has become abundant. Like I said, the hunter-gatherers eating patterns didn't follow breakfast-lunch-and-dinner but were completely random. Faunal mobility, seasonal change and drought all determined whether or not they would have to fast or feast. On top of that, there were sabertooth tigers whose dinner they could've easily become themselves.

Everything in the past was uncertain and unpredictable. Now it's less so. We expect things to happen and our intuition is to stick to a certain regimen. We want to wake up every morning in our safe bed, go through our daily routines and go back to sleep the same way.

It's in our nature to want to avoid change because any deviation from homeostasis forces us to exert more energy and makes us adapt to novelty. We're slaves to our habits and want things to happen exactly the way we want them to.

Despite our hardest efforts, what's certain is that the only constant is change. Uncertainty is an innate part of the conduct of the cosmos. We can never be completely sure what's going to happen to us next.

Rest assured, the likelihood of the highly improbable asserts that *sh*t will hit the fan* sooner or later. Things will never stay the same and after every upside there is inevitably going to be a downfall, like with insulin. Once that occurs we'll be dumbstruck and incapable of handling it.

The more conditioned you are in dealing with random events, the stronger you'll be as an organism. *Antifragility* is the term coined by Nassim Nicholas Taleb, that describes this. He has also written a book on the subject titled *Antifragile: Things That Gain From Disorder.* Prepare yourself, because this chapter will now enter into a deep philosophical rabbit hole from which I'm not sure we'll recover from completely.

Taleb introduces the book as: *"Some things benefit from shocks; they thrive and grow when exposed to volatility, randomness, disorder, and stressors and love adventure, risk, and uncertainty. Yet, in spite of the ubiquity of the phenomenon, there is no word for the exact opposite of fragile. Let us call it antifragile. Antifragility is beyond resilience or robustness. The resilient resists shocks and stays the same; the antifragile gets better."*

Hormesis is an example of antifragility that increases the resilience of our organism. Intermittent fasting is a stressor that contributes to growth by stimulating destruction. It's like the phoenix that burns itself with its feathers and then rises from the ashes, more magnificent than ever before.

Taleb continues by defining the phenomenon as a non-linear response: *"Simply, antifragility is defined as a convex response to a stressor or source of harm (for some range of variation), leading to a positive sensitivity to increase in volatility (or variability, stress, dispersion of outcomes, or uncertainty, what is grouped under the designation "disorder cluster"). Likewise, fragility is defined as a concave sensitivity to stressors, leading a negative sensitivity to increase in volatility. The relation between fragility, convexity and sensitivity to disorder is mathematical, obtained by theorem, not derived from empirical data mining or some historical narrative. It is a priori"*

A priori is a Latin phrase coined by the philosopher Immanuel Kant, meaning *"from the earlier."* It's knowledge or justification about something that's independent of experience (2+2=4 and *All bachelors are unmarried*) – it's objective truth.

A posteriori, meaning *"from the latter"*, is the opposite, based on experience and empirical evidence, as is the case with most fields of science and our own personal knowledge. It's about predicting an outcome by relying on what has happened before us and is thus fragile because the past is never the same as the present.

The eating patterns of hunter-gatherers made them *antifragile*. Our body actually gets stronger and more resilient at times of scarcity and stress. The response that gets created triggers hormonal and physiological effects, that lead to beneficial and empowering adaptations.

On the flip side, the constant feeding in the modern society makes us more fragile. We become more dependent of food, as is shown by the increased hunger and slothfulness it causes. Frequent eating conditions our body to be weaker when there are no calories around.

In Taleb's earlier book *The Black Swan: The Impact of the Highly Improbable* he describes 2 models of distribution types for unexpected events.

- Mediocristan is where normal things happen, where they're expected, and have low impact. The bell curve and normal distribution are great examples of this. Any single phenomenon or individual will represent only a small part of the total. For example, height, weight and your caloric intake are in this realm. If you take a few hundred people, there is no human whose height significantly differs from the average. You won't meet someone who is a 1000 feet tall. Low-impact changes have the highest chances of occurring, and huge, wide-impact ones have a very small probability.

- Extremistan is a different place. There nothing can be predicted with great accuracy and unlikely, seemingly impossible, events occur frequently and have a huge impact. One single observation or event can completely disrupt the outcome. Imagine a room full of 30 random people. If you calculated the average of their salary, the odds are the average would seem pretty reasonable. However, if you added Bill Gates to the room and then do it again, your average would jump up by a huge margin. One individual would comprise more than 90% of the total draft. Book sales, viral videos and 911 type of accidents are all from Extremistan.

What does it have to do with this book?

Mediocristan is what natural, biological evolution looks like and functions. It's a system with moderate and gradual variation. Our caloric intake belongs here as well. No matter how much you eat at Christmas Eve, you can't double your weight in a single day. This is the realm, in which the 99.5% of the world lives in.

Non-biological man-made systems, such as business, finance etc. live in much harsher conditions, in Extremistan. Single events have changed history, such as the storming of Bastille and World War I. Sudden, explosive, violent, irreversible. Most of all, unforeseen.

With the development of technology, we'll be moving further into Extremistan, but we still think we're in Mediocristan. It's going to be a winner-takes all effect. If you stand around wondering who the *sucker* is, then look no further – it's you.

The famous example Taleb uses in his book is the Thanksgiving turkey. *"Consider a turkey that is fed every day. Every single feeding will firm up the bird's belief that it is the general rule of life to be fed every day by friendly members of the human race 'looking out for its best interests,' as a politician would say. On the afternoon of the Wednesday before Thanksgiving, something unexpected will happen to the turkey. It will incur a revision of belief."* We all know what people eat at Thanksgiving dinner, and that butchers are especially busy during holidays.

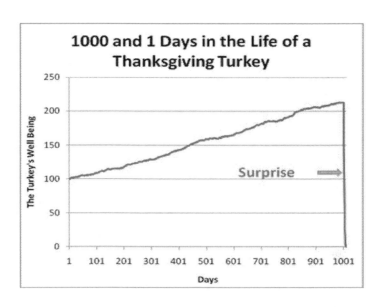

1000 and 1 Days in the Life of a Thanksgiving Turkey

Surprise ➡

The Turkey's Well Being (y-axis: 0, 50, 100, 150, 200, 250)

Days (x-axis: 1, 101, 201, 301, 401, 501, 601, 701, 801, 901, 1001)

"But the problem is even more general than that; it strikes at the nature of empirical knowledge itself. Something has worked in the past, until — well, it unexpectedly no longer does, and what we have learned from the past turns out to be at best irrelevant or false, at worst viciously misleading," - Taleb continues.

It's foolish to base our future forecasts a _posteriori_ because it predisposes us to be dependent of events that have happened in the past. Our mind will always default to this mode and expects things to stay the same because it likes comfort. First rule of Extremistan: _"Don't be a turkey."_

By the same token, for something to have a significant impact, it needs to be a Black Swan. This applies to physiological adaptations as well. Evolution happens gradually, but in order for something to take affect it needs to be instigated by something powerful. You don't get stronger by lifting a pillow off the ground millions of times. On the flip side, deadlift 400 pounds only for a few repetitions and you get a much greater response.

Even though our BMR is in Mediocristan, the eating patterns of hunter-gatherers were still more on the side of Extremistan, between feasting and fasting. Both are distinctive ends of the spectrum. There wasn't any set time schedule for their meals and they were thus *antifragile*.

Practices like stoicism and intermittent fasting are strategies of *antifragility*. It doesn't matter what happens to us – we'll still benefit from it. That's why Seneca is considered to be one of the most influential writers in this school of philosophy.

Fasting keeps those vital pathways alive and well embedded into our physiology. Instead of being negatively influenced by unpredictable events, we get stronger and better. Even when there's no direct necessity for it at the moment, we're still being very vulnerable to change. You can make all the grandiose plans you'd like, but it only takes a tiny bit of randomness to topple even the highest of skyscrapers.

Complete randomness is, by virtue, complete randomness. What about *controlled randomness* - deliberate carving of oneself into *antifragility*. That could work.

There's less uncertainty in our society across all domains, aside from Black Swans flying in from Extremistan into the World Trading Center, but most definitely in our eating patterns. Deliberate intermittent fasting is like controlled randomness - we create it almost artificially and voluntarily embrace change. It's like throwing spokes inside our own wheels, which will force us to adapt.

You voluntarily seek out novel stimuli that can't be predicted and will cause uncertain events to occur. However, the results can be predicted because of your competence, to a certain degree of course. That's as close you can get to becoming a seer. Not being able to tell the future *per se*, but to know that you're more than capable of handling any change.

There's still going to be an invisible safety net around you, as there's food everywhere you look. You're not going to starve to death even when you try very hard. Here lies the intentional aspect of it. Rather than being subject to circumstance, you rise above it and make your own terms with the environment.

Let me share with you a scene from an international airport. People are waiting for their flight and have to spend hours sitting at cafeterias. There's not much to do – they're bored and eventually get frustrated. Those who break sooner than others give in to their hunger and start searching for something to eat.

It's like the savannah – they have to be on the lookout and it's as if they're stalking for prey. The only exception is that their meal is certain - they only have to make a decision. There's too much to choose from and none of them are any good. Airport food is unhealthy and filled with empty calories that give us no actual energy and only light up our taste buds. *"But you have* to eat something..." is the most common excuse. Based on this book, there's no actual physiological reason for doing so, unless your flight is to Mars.

They want to eat to satisfy their psychological hunger, alleviate boredom and to reinforce their habits of meal timing. Their body is already expecting for food because the same thing happens at the exact time every single day. Instead of not being influenced by this random course of events, they're fragile and fall on the ground into millions of pieces.

Me, as I'm looking at this, have been fasting for 24 hours and will continue to do so. I've also carried my baggage of 30 kilos with me the entire day and yet don't feel any worse off because of that. This has no significant impact on me, as I'm used to being used to uncertainty. To be honest, I'm gaining from the situation, as it's the perfect time for being productive and getting things done.

Looking back, I think that some of my antifragility came from my time in the military. In fact, I'm a certified sniper and a sharpshooter. This is probably the most uncertain vocations in the army. You can never be sure how much time you're going to spend out in the field or what you might come across. Sometimes you had to be in one spot to conduct observation for hours. At others you had to walk through knee deep swamps behind enemy lines. The few snacks you can fit into your pocket will run out very quickly, so it is with water. There had been countless occasions where our company's supply team had forgotten to include us into their rations and we went hungry. *Very funny guys...* Nevertheless, we thrived – we clenched our teeth and endured.

That's why I would recommend doing different types of intermittent fasting. The majority of your day should still be spent fasted because of the hormonal effects, but try bringing in as much variety to when you eat. Instead of following a strict schedule all the time, let the waves of life hit you right in the face and adjust to the flow of them. When you don't have the opportunity to break your fast the way you wanted to don't feel frustrated about it and embrace being *antifragile*. It's a great power to have.

Chapter IX

Fasting and Feasting

Like I said, it doesn't matter what type of intermittent fasting you do as long as you simply do it. Here's where I'm going to show you the protocol of this book. The reasoning behind every action and timing of our food intake is based on objectivity and doing things as optimally as possible.

To get the most benefit from daily intermittent fasting, I would recommend you to push your breakfast past noon and spend the majority of the day in an underfed state. Even your first meal should be as low in calories as possible so that your body would remain slightly hungry.

The minimum I would recommend is 14 hours of fasting. 16 is a good point and you don't really have to go any longer than that, if you do it every day. However, occasionally going past the 20-hour mark is very empowering.

The hormonal and hormetic response will be immense and your body will actually get stronger. What makes it all work is that you'll be eating at dinner – overfeeding, to be honest. Hence the name of this book. During the day you'll be fasting like a beast and at night feasting like a king.

Your body will perceive the slight starvation signal as a threat and will maximize food utilization and protein synthesis.

The same adaptations occur with resistance training. If you lifted 400 pounds last week, then your muscles will expect you to encounter even more force in the future. As a result, you'll get stronger because it's conditioned by your environment. In the case of antifragility, you know that things are uncertain, or that *sh*t will hit the fan,* but you're anticipating it to happen and aren't negatively influenced by it. Your body isn't dependent of food and can still produce energy without the presence of exogenous calories because it's so used to being underfed.

If done properly then it won't actually feel like an abstention from food and becomes incredibly enjoyable. With no hunger you can hardly tell or feel that you haven't eaten. You'll be completely satiated because of being able to tap into your fuel tank with infinite potentiality.

Here are the best tips and things to remember that will make fasting incredibly easy.

- **Drink a lot of water.** Most of the time people get hungry not because they need to eat but because they're actually dehydrated. Instead of quitting half-way through, have a glass of water and wait for 15 minutes. Once you've absorbed the aqua, the feeling of hunger will go away. Sparkling water is a possibility as the carbonation usually decreases appetite. Also, you don't want an additional stressor on the body and become dehydrated. Mineral water would be ideal as the electrolytes and salts will decrease cortisol. Drink lots of it, as it will cleanse you at the same time. The minimum should be at least half a gallon or 2 liters but more is advisable, especially during your undereating phase. To reduce the stress response of fasting and keep your adrenals from getting overstimulated, have a big glass of water with a teaspoon of sea salt mixed into it first thing in the morning.

- **Non-caloric beverages.** To maintain a fasted state, we need to avoid consuming calories. This doesn't mean that we can't drink some tea or coffee. Don't add any sugar, cream or milk though. Have it black. One thing to remember is to not become dependent of them. Coffee decreases appetite but at the same time dehydrates us. Stick to only a maximum of 2-4 cups a day and resort to it only when hunger kicks in. Don't drink it first thing in the morning either and wait a few hours. If you're not hungry then you don't need to cash in on this powerful stimulant. You'll have a back-up card to draw upon once you need it. Green tea gets a green light. Avoid diet-sodas as well despite their non-caloric content. The artificial sweeteners still give rise to blood sugar, creating a placebo-like fed state. You don't want to release insulin for nothing.

- **Brush your teeth.** This can help you reduce hunger. There may be some artificial sweeteners in your tooth paste so be wary. You should use it as a last resort or when you don't want to drink coffee. Sugar free chewing gum is fine as well. However, it has some calories in it. Don't eat more than 2-3 pieces. Overall, it refreshes your mouth and makes your breath smell really nice.

- **Apple cider vinegar.** It's mainly used for household and cooking purposes. What you maybe don't know is that it also has powerful health benefits. Lower blood sugar levels, better fat loss and improved symptoms of diabetes. Its biological components are very effective and acidic, that can be good for digestion sometimes. By the same token, it will also destroy bad bacteria in your gut and make you less hungry. You can add it to salads or other food during your feeding window. While fasting, get a glass of warm water and add 1-2 teaspoons of apple cider vinegar. Any more than that may have some unwanted consequences, so don't go overboard. Consume it right away and be done with it. Your body will thank you.

- **Keep your mind busy.** One of the biggest reasons why people eat so often is because they're bored. When I'm fasting I get the majority of my creative endeavors done. While focusing on something else, other than the fact that I'm fasting, then time will pass by without me even noticing that I haven't eaten. If you make a big deal out of it, then you'll inevitably get hungry and groggy. Also, it's a great opportunity to reap the benefits of mental clarity and improved concentration. During those morning hours of fasting my mind is sharp as a knife and can easily cut through any intellectual problem I might come face to face with. Not that I couldn't do it at any other time. It's just that when not having to digest food we can allocate our mental resources to much more important things. Additionally, meditating over it is another great option. Sit down and become mindful of how your body is reacting. It's quite an interesting experience.

- **Move around.** Despite the fact that we're in a fasted state it doesn't mean we should avoid moving our bodies. The initial response might be to preserve energy and stay on the couch. However, doing so would only promote slothfulness and is another way to make a big deal out of fasting. For hunter-gatherers, survival depended on those moments. They wouldn't have got to tell an excuse to their prey that they haven't eaten for a while and would like the animal to voluntarily offer itself to be killed. It doesn't work like that. Instead, they still had to exert themselves during the hunt and had to do so even more than normally. If they would miss an opportunity, then they would have to suffer even longer. Therefore, there was no room for failure. We don't have to go through the same strenuous process. Going for a walk is not just the best way of getting more movement into our day but also gets the mind out of its own rut. Intense training is also an opportunity as the hormonal benefits would be especially evident afterwards. For instance, occasionally I fast for 20 hours, have a hard workout, wait for a few hours and then have my first meal. I'm able to do so because I'm so used to fasting by now and my ketogenic pathways are very deep. What's best is that I don't experience any difference in blood pressure or faintness. That's the way we're supposed to feel even after shortly exercising. It's an incredibly empowering *antifragile* ability.

- **Don't make a big deal out of it.** During my first experimental 24 hour fast I realized that the sensation of hunger and weakness is only an illusion. If I thought about the fact that I hadn't been eating for over 20 hours, I immediately began to feel bad. However, by telling myself that it's nothing special everything got better, actually wonderful. It's really an interesting experience. For me, I become more mindful of my blood flow and muscle contraction. During that time one will definitely get more in touch with their body.

- **Write about your experience.** If you're doing fasts that last for longer than a day, then I definitely advise you to document it in some shape or form. It helps you to reflect back on what you may have missed and also takes some pressure off your mind. You can get a notebook or video record yourself.

I've also used some breathing techniques during my fasting, which would reduce hunger and make the entire process more illuminating. Deep nasal breathing into your abdomen stimulates the parasympathetic nervous system and reduces stress. It's a great way to voluntarily control your autonomic nervous system.

Simply inhale deeply, starting from the bottom of your stomach and reaching the top of your lungs. Exhale the same way and do it for a few minutes. This will also massage your intestines and improves digestion.

We should all pay more attention to our breathing, as it's the most direct way our nervous system experiences the world. If we're gasping for air or doing shallow mouth-breathing, then the body will perceive the environment as dangerous, whereas in reality you're safely inside your house. Being mindful of your respiratory process enables you to become aware of what goes on inside you and increases your consciousness.

While fasting, there are several therapeutic measures that can be taken to enhance the cleansing and detoxification process. Here are a few examples.

- **Anointing, oleation, oil massage**. Massaging the entire body with fragrant medicated oils improves the circulation and detoxification of blood and lymph. It also increases the dumping of waste materials into the gastrointestinal tract for elimination.

- **Castor oil.** An amazing detoxifier because it draws out toxins. Drink one to two tablespoons, flushed down with lemon water, to cleanse the bowels at night before going to sleep, or massage into the abdomen and pelvis to loosen up the bowels. Massaging it into the liver and gall bladder areas will ease purification crises.

- **Clay** is a mineral with a negative ionic charge, which chelates and draws out positively charged acidic toxins. Before you use it soak it in some water for a couple of hours to ionize it properly. If you want to drink it, then mix about a few pinches to a quarter teaspoon of dry powdered clay into a cup of water and let it stand for a while. Clay paste can also be applied to rashes, boils and other skin eruptions to draw out toxins and hasten recovery.

- **Herbal teas.** Different herb teas help the body in cleaning and detoxifying. Since you're already fasting, it's better not to take strongly eliminative or purgative herbs. Use simple and gentle ones, such as lemongrass, ginger, dandelion, milk thistle, green and black teas.

- **Enemas and colonics.** Cleansing the colon might seem nasty, but it's an ancient practice and a good idea. On longer fasts, it prevents toxins from old fecal matter from being reabsorbed into the body. Coffee enemas are said to also be very healthy and cleansing. I'm not going to tell you how to do it, and if you're interested, then you should seek out a professional.

- **Sweating** is another inner body mechanism that excretes toxins. It's our skins natural response to heat that detoxifies the pours and keeps the blood circulating. We should engage in some sweaty activities on a daily basis, even when we're not fasting. Doing Bikram yoga and taking a sauna are great ways for conducting these natural purification processes.

Getting used to undereating takes time. Our body adapts to exactly the environment it gets exposed to. Give it frequent eating in conjunction with snacking and you'll be more parasympathetic dominant. Fast and you'll set yourself up for increased resistance to stress and less hunger.

How does it feel like going for several days without eating? To be honest, there isn't much difference. The deeper you get into ketosis, the less of an effect it will have. Most of the time I feel just the same as I do on a ketogenic menu. The only thing is that you get more cautious, if that would be the right word to describe it, because of your body wanting to preserve energy. You almost go into a conservation mode in which you're unconsciously trying not to exert yourself. This, and having occasional brief hunger that shortly disappears.

The response that gets created is caused by habitual conditioning. You have to do it to a certain extent every day. Every function of an organism is there for a reason. If your muscles don't encounter resistance, then they won't grow. The same thing applies to your ketogenic pathways. What you don't use, you'll lose.

How to Break Your Fast

When you break your fast, the immediate reaction of our urges would be to eat everything in sight. Don't gorge afterwards. If you've mustered enough self-mastery to make it this far, then it shouldn't be a problem to control yourself just a little bit longer. The body needs time to readjust to food and eating a heavy meal right away would put too much stress on the intestines.

Instead, what we need to do is slowly ease into it. The best way to start off is with a glass of hot lemon water. The citric acid gets absorbed really quickly and promotes the production of good digestive enzymes in the gut. This will wake up the intestines and prepares them for the feasting that's to come.

Your first meal should be something small and low-glycemic. This will keep you in a semi-fasted state because of the non-existent rise in blood sugar. Carbohydrate refeeding after fasting causes an abrupt weight gain[xlii]. A spike of insulin will help you shuttle nutrients into your cells but also has some negative side-effects.

It's probably the reason why the majority of civilization has become so slothful. After the agricultural revolution, man started consuming refined grains, eating more often and avoiding intense physical movement. Carbs make you tired, slow and mentally dull, whereas a diet of more protein, fat and vegetables keeps your muscles tense, body toned and mind sharp as a knife.

After you break the fast wait about 1-2 hours and have your biggest meal of the day. Because you'll be consuming the majority of your calories at dinner, it's going to be quite the feast. Depending on your condition, you'll be easily consuming about 2000 calories within a few hours. It wouldn't be difficult to go even beyond that either.

This is the overfeeding phase that flips the switch from catabolism to ultimate anabolism. Your body will supercompensate for all of the hormetic responses and starts to repair itself. All of the nutrients you consume will be utilized a lot more efficiently and protein synthesis speeds up.

It's thought that you can only absorb about 30 grams of protein per meal. In the case of 6 meals a day it might be true but because of the period of underfeeding, our body will be more readily available to use it. What's more is that ketosis reduces muscle catabolism and prevents the loss of lean tissue thanks to the increased utilization of ketones.

Amino acids and some peptides are able to self-regulate their time in the intestines. For example, the digestive hormone CCK can slow down intestinal contractions and speed in response to protein [xliii]. It gets released in the presence of dietary protein and slows down digestion to absorb all of those nutrients [xliv].

Our intestines will contract according to the speed at which it can digest food. If they can't handle any more protein, then they won't waste this precious resource away but will store it. After a few moments it will continue absorption. This happens because the body won't be able to supercompensate without overfeeding itself. It wants to repair the damage and is willing to do whatever it takes to grow.

A single high protein meal can actually be more effective because of that. Intermittent fasting studies show that there is no difference in lean mass gain by consuming 80-100 grams of protein in 4 hours, in comparison to more frequent eating [xlv].

Before you eat, take a moment to step back and reflect on the experience. First of all, you realize that fasting isn't a big deal and instead very good for us. Secondly, you should be thankful for having a meal. Most people forget about how fortunate it is to have food around and they become mindless about what they consume.

By doing occasional intermittent fasting every meal becomes more appreciated. Family dinners turn into feasts where eating not only becomes more meaningful but the entire atmosphere improves. Everything, even bland food, becomes tastier as our taste buds have managed to become free from the constantly stimulating effect of refined carbohydrates and sugar.

What's most important, you realize that you don't need to be eating every few hours and can thus accept nothing less than optimal nutrition. Mindless eating in a rush becomes a thing of the past as we teach our body to always have abundant energy readily available.

Chapter X

How to Do Intermittent Fasting, IF...

There are different reasons why we should do intermittent fasting. For me, it's not about caloric restriction or weight loss. I actually consume as much food as I would on a normal eating schedule. It's just that the controlled periods of undereating and overfeeding have too many benefits for me to pass out on.

By manipulating our hormones and deliberately stimulating our physiology in a certain way we're causing specific adaptations to occur inside the body. Because of being conscious enough, us humans are aware of these metabolic processes and can voluntarily control them according to our liking. It's like mastering our own biology.

But there are also different scenarios we can use intermittent fasting for. First and foremost, IF is a very effective tool for fat loss. At the same time, you can build muscle and strength with it as well.

Let's go through all of the situations.

...You Want to Burn Fat

The first law of thermodynamics dictates weight loss or gain. Calories in versus calories out determine body composition. Basically, you can eat whatever you want and lose fat, as long as you stay at a negative energy balance.

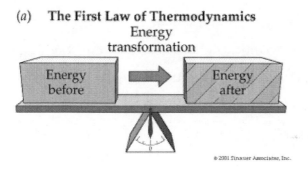

(a) The First Law of Thermodynamics
Energy
transformation

© 2001 Sinauer Associates, Inc.

However, weight loss doesn't necessarily equal fat loss. Nutrition influences our hormones, which have a much more profound impact on our health and longevity. You don't want your body to solely break down its valuable tissue. Instead, you want it to happen safely.

Why do some people mainly lose muscle and not fat? Because they're not efficient enough with using stored calories as fuel. That's why you need to practice some form of intermittent fasting, so that your body wouldn't become too dependent of food for energy.

If your main purpose is to burn as much fat as possible and not build muscle or get stronger, then the best strategy would be to do the 24-hour fast daily. This will almost by default put you into a caloric deficit and makes it very easy to maintain. You'll still be able to enjoy delicious food while staying in a negative energy balance. What's best about it is that once you get used to it you'll be extremely satiated with only 1 meal a day and don't feel the need to overeat, as some may fear.

Intermittent fasting is a much more reasonable way to create a negative energy balance than exercising. Doing long hours of cardio is actually bad for us as the repetitive motion induces too much stress on our adrenals and damage to the joints. What's more, it doesn't even work as well as you think it does.

Doing 10 minutes of steady state cardio burns about 100 calories. Now, one single banana has about as many calories. Would it be easier to not eat it in the first place? Even worse, one slice of pizza and a can of soda has about 600 calories, which you can consume in less than 5 minutes.

Exercise is 1 step forward in the right direction. But a poor diet is 2 steps back. Simply put, you can't out-exercise bad nutrition. It's the treadmill effect – you have to keep trying harder and harder to keep yourself at one spot. You just have to keep on running and running, otherwise the ground beneath you will wipe you off. No matter how many hours you spend rolling inside the wheel like a hamster, you'll never reach your results if you make it all go down the drain.

The root cause here is desire – you want to eat copious amounts of food and are solely attached to it. This is what the Buddhist monks have realized as well. Desire creates cravings and causes suffering, as you'll never be satisfied enough. You'll keep on wanting for something you currently don't have. This is another problem of our society – we're too materialistic and are chasing possessions one after another. Once you become more conscious and rid yourself from the desire, you'll reach your outcome because you've achieved freedom from the outcome.

Only people who lack self-mastery gorge themselves. They're driven by their scavenger mentality and can't control their subconscious urges. They might be aware of the presence of these processes but they still can't assert their dominance. In that case, you would have to first spend some time thinking about how big of an effect food has on you and what kind of a relationship you want to create.

Follow me on yet another mind trip. Sit down and close your eyes. Become completely present and centered. Think about your life. Where are, what are you doing every day and who are the people you're surrounded by? Whatever the situation might be, express your gratitude, as it can definitely be worse. Understand that food shouldn't be something that makes you happy *per se* but improves the quality of your living. It's not foundational but a great addition. It's not going to be your last meal and there's an abundance of food for everyone. Scarcity is nowhere to be found.

Becoming more conscious as a person is very important. Practices of mindfulness will not only make you savor food a lot more but will also help you in understanding your physiology and psychology better.

How much food should you eat?

Well, it would depend on your total daily energy expenditure (TDEE). This includes our basal metabolic rate (BMR) and our activity levels.

Use these simple formulas to calculate your basal metabolic rate (BMR). This is the number which we would have to consume by doing nothing – simply breathing and lying in bed.

- **Imperial system.**

  - Women: BMR=655 + (4.35 x weight in pounds) + (4.7 x height in inches) - (4.7 x age in years)

  - Men: BMR = 66 + (6.23 x weight in pounds) + (12.7 x height in inches) - (6.8 x age in year)

- **Metric system.**

  - Women: BMR = 655 + (9.6 x weight in kilos) + (1.8 x height in cm) - (4.7 x age in years)

  - Men: BMR = 66 + (13.7 x weight in kilos) + (5 x height in cm) - (6.8 x age in years)

What adds onto it are our activity levels - how much we move around, how often and at what intensity. That's why an athlete needs more calories than a sedentary person would because they're constantly using energy.

Our actual caloric requirements need to be derived from personal experience. We can't rely on our own predictions on how much we've burned. The number won't actually dictate energy balance as there are other factors involved.

No formula will tell us exactly how much we've burned and it would be unreasonable as well. Simply going through a lot of trial and error will show us how much we habitually need. By gaining weight we're in the positive and if we're losing then we're in the negative.

To steadily lose fat, you would have to have a negative energy balance of about 500-700 calories. You can even go up to a 1000 but should only do so for a short period. Your BMR will drop in response to caloric restriction, because of the body wanting to hold onto as much back up storage as possible. To mitigate that, you should also consider eating at maintenance after a few days of dieting. Too aggressive deficits aren't sustainable and can cause metabolic damage. Additionally, you can have one or two 24-hour fasts a week and eat normally rest of the days. Patience is a virtue.

If you want to burn fat as fast as possible then restricting your carbohydrate intake is a good idea. Your body won't start burning fat at an accelerated rate until it's endogenous glucose tank has been depleted. It's like trying to out-exercise yourself again. Once your glycogen stores have run out, you'll start using more ketone bodies as fuel. Any deficit you have will come straight from the adipose tissue. The ketogenic diet is extremely effective for this.

You can be quite meticulous, but counting calories isn't necessary. Of course, you won't be able to burn fat while staying at a caloric surplus. It's just that by having only 1 meal a day you'll simply be so satisfied that you don't feel the need to eat any more.

To promote fat burning you can create an even larger calorie deficit by training before overfeeding. Fasted workouts increase fat oxidation even further. Aerobic exercise in a fasted state increases your use of fatty acids[xlvi]., because of the body being in a state of mild ketosis but isn't detrimental. This happens because your liver glycogen stores are empty after an overnight fast. If you follow a ketogenic diet, then it doesn't matter when you train. At the end of the day, it's still about a negative caloric balance.

To lose fat and keep it off, it's best advised to do resistance training instead. Cardio burns calories and increases our TDEE, but building muscle adds onto our BMR, which is a lot more powerful. It's easier to put more default energy demands on your body than it is to constantly run on a treadmill like a hamster inside a wheel. It will also stimulate anabolic growth once you enter the overfeeding phase.

Compound movements that tax the body as a whole are the best for doing this. Squats, deadlifts, bench pressing, overhead pressing and pull-ups cause significant hormonal responses. Bodyweight equivalents include handstand push-ups, pistol squats, front levers etc. They're also the most *antifragile* of exercises.

The rep/set scheme isn't as important but there is some common consensus. Strength is built most with lower reps at about 2-6, hypertrophy (muscle size) increases between 6-12 and anything beyond that contributes mainly to endurance.

The less reps you do the more sets you need to create an adequate stimulus. In total, you should aim for about 20-30 reps per exercise. If you do 8 reps, then go for 3 sets etc. Train for at least 3-4 times a week and you'll get incredibly fit and strong. Aerobic cardio isn't bad for you, it just shouldn't be our main focus.

What gets neglected most is simple walking. It's the best form of exercise, as it doesn't tax our body at all and keeps us on the move. Instead of going to the gym to punish yourself all the time, it's a lot better idea to simply walk in nature. I would recommend you walk for at least 30-60 minutes a day. It actually causes very good adaptations, just like training does.

...*You Want to Build Muscle*

Fitness gurus want you to believe that you need to eat 6 small meals a day. On top of that, you need to have a pre-workout, intra-workout and post-workout protein shake. Otherwise you'll be burning muscle. Yes, that seems reasonable, if you have a line of supplements to sell to people.

Meal timing is not significant when it comes to body composition. At least amongst the majority of people. Only bodybuilders who are on steroids need to eat very often so that they could promote their unnatural muscle mass. The same goes for *elite level athletes* who are training many hours per day. No offence, but most of us don't workout like Michael Phelps or Ronnie Coleman.

I've been able to build muscle and gain strength while still sticking to intermittent fasting. What stimulates growth isn't the food you eat but the resistance of training. Eating enough protein and calories simply enhances that process. At the end of the day, what determines weight gain is a positive energy balance.

Intermittent fasting is also practiced by Hugh Jackman. In preparation for his role as Wolverine, he would train intensely about 3 hours a day and eat a ton of food during his 8 hour feeding window. He was able to build muscle and burn fat like crazy - all thanks to IF. Whenever I hear other celebrities talking about how they starve themselves by eating 6 meals of chicken breast and broccoli a day to get fit, I always shake my head in disbelief. How come they think that there isn't a better way?

The missing piece of the puzzle that gets overlooked is adequate hormonal output. To build muscle you need mainly testosterone and HGH. On top of that, insulin and IGF-1 are relevant and influential but not necessary.

As we've already discussed, fasting induces ketosis, which is a metabolic state that preserves muscle mass and decreases the use of glycogen at the expense of ketones. HGH also gets skyrocketed to outer space. An increase of 1300-2000% is still mind-blowing to me.

This makes perfect sense, as a hunter-gatherer wouldn't have managed to survive times of scarcity if all the body did was cannibalize its own tissue. To chase mammoths, spear saber-tooth tigers and wrestle bears, you would have to have a lot of strength and endurance. In order to survive in the dangerous environment of the Paleolithic, our ancestors had to be world class athletes capable of performing in any situation under any circumstances. Lean muscle is invaluable for the success of hunting and the body will find ways of maintaining it, especially at times when there's no food around.

All of the anabolic hormones get stimulated by fasting. Training fasted may actually boost the post-workout response more favorably than doing it in a fed-state [xlvii]. The reason why some hard gainers might not be able to put on muscle is that their body is simply conditioned to be lazy and doesn't know how to use its internal energy sources. You need to first be catabolic before you can be effectively anabolic.

Using intermittent fasting to build muscle promotes longevity as well. One of the muscle building pathways is mTOR (mammalian target of rapamycin). But it's a double-edged sword, as it's also associated with cancer and tumor growth. It's essential for getting stronger and more muscular, but having it elevated all of the time isn't a good idea for obvious reasons. That's probably why some bodybuilders who are anabolic almost 24/7, thanks to taking steroids and consuming excessive amounts of protein, die a premature death (R.I.P. Zyzz, the son of Zeus). I don't think vanity is worth having an early grave.

Exercise, intermittent fasting and protein fasting inhibit mTOR expression for a brief period, which will then have a rebound effect once you start eating again. Overfeeding is highly anabolic, but it lasts only for a short amount of time. At other times, when in a fasted state, we're increasing our lifespan and fighting the spreading of disease thanks to the rise in growth hormone and increased *autophagy*.

Building muscle with intermittent fasting is easy and you can do so without gaining excess body fat. You'll actually be building primarily lean tissue, as the majority of the day you'll be burning ketones. There isn't a need to bulk up and get fat in the process. You simply have to be in a small caloric surplus (about 500) and gradually get stronger and more built.

In this case, you would also want to reduce your fasting window. The 16/8 formula is perfect for some lean gains, as prescribed by Martin Berkhan. A small meal at lunch will add an extra period of protein synthesis, which will yield augmenting effects. You don't really need to eat any more than 2 times a day, if you want to get more muscular.

If you workout fasted, then your post-workout meal should be your biggest meal of the day. If you choose to eat something before, then keep your fast-breaking food intake as small as possible. You still want to be underfed and mildly ketogenic during training because it causes more anabolic growth afterwards.

What causes muscle growth in the first place is an adequate training stimulus. You need to workout hard enough to force your body to adapt to the resistance. Even a 3-day fast has no negative effect on how strong you can contract your muscles[xlviii], your ability to do short term high intensity or longer periods of moderate exercise.

The need to eat before an intense workout is mainly psychological. Ori Hofmekler says in his book *The Warrior Diet: "Predators in the wild only hunt when they are hungry."* What's stopping you is your own mind.

Breaking personal records in training may be difficult, especially when you're fasted. However, the more you practice this, the better you get at it. The first sets will definitely be more exerting than you would've thought, but once you warm up you'll unleash your inner predator.

Whatever the case might be, I would still recommend pushing your meals as late into the day as possible. Of course, you don't want to be consuming 2000+ calories an hour before bed.

You'll be bloated and constipated. The overfeeding window lasts for several hours and can consist of many meals.

The best time to workout is after 4PM. According to the circadian rhythm, our strength and agility will be at their peak. What's more, if we've spent the day undereating, insulin sensitivity will be a lot higher at about 7PM as well. That's the perfect time for dinner.

To build lean muscle you don't need to eat over a 500 calorie surplus. Anything higher than that will create a point of diminishing returns and causes unnecessary fat gain. Dirty bulking is just another excuse for eating junk food. You have to make sure you train hard enough in the first place.

Additionally, your minimum daily protein intake should be at about 0.7g-1.4g per lean body mass. There is no reason to go any higher than that, as the excess will simply be converted to sugar. Only bodybuilders on steroids need to have 24-hour protein synthesis to support their size. That's just not achievable naturally, nor is it healthy.

...*You Are a Woman.*

Now, I'm not trying to enforce some sort of an inequality between genders, but in the case of nutrition there are some differences.

Fasting ketosis develops more rapidly in women than in men[xlix]. Serum FFA and ketone levels increase at a greater rate as well[l]. Reasons might be higher glucagon levels, which have been shown to be higher in non-obese women than in men[li], estrogen effects and differential conversion of FFAs to ketone bodies[lii].

A common misconception concerning fasting is that it decreases fertility in women and testosterone in men. This happens only when you're already at a very low body fat. If you're getting enough calories during your overfeeding phase, then it shouldn't be an issue.

Based on that, it would seem that women do better in a fasted state. However, IF may cause some hormonal imbalances in women, because they're more sensitive to starvation signals.

Evolutionarily, it's more important for them to keep their ovaries and fertility in check, because one egg is more valuable than millions of sperm cells.

I wouldn't recommend fasting for pregnant women, women who are breastfeeding, extremely underweight, or very young (<16-years old). Everyone else can only potentially gain from it. If you have some sort of a severe medical condition, then I would advise you to consult your physician first. Chances are they'll put you on drugs and a low-fat diet instead. That's going to work just fine...

If intermittent fasting is done daily, then the fast should be reduced to the 14-hour mark. In the case of *Eat Stop Eat* or *Alternate Day Fasting* type of dieting, then you can follow the prescribed methods. It's just that the stimulus of fasting will become too strong, if done too often.

Chapter XI

First Fast, Then Feast

This book is about fasting, but it's also about feasting. During the undereating phase we'll be only consuming water or other non-caloric beverages. But what about the overfeeding? What should we eat for dinner?

There isn't much I can do to change your eating preferences. Everything is an acquired taste and we like to eat just that what we're habitually used to consuming. I myself follow a low carb ketogenic diet.

Whatever your goals might be, it's obvious that whole Paleo-type foods are most optimal. For body composition you can eat anything you'd like, but calories in versus calories out doesn't include health and longevity.

We're supposed to do deliberate intermittent fasting not solely to burn fat or build muscle but for the other physiological effects we get, such as increased hormonal response, *autophagy* and longevity. It's meant to enhance the quality of our relationship with food and overall life.

There are still some general guidelines I would recommend everyone follow.

It's clear that while fasting you shouldn't consume any calories. The undereating phase will continue once you have your first meal. It should be something low glycemic and not very high in calories. Some protein and fat with fibrous vegetables will keep you satiated for long. If you eat a lot of carbs and sugar right away, you'll create more cravings. By not spiking your blood sugar levels right away, you will actually mimic fasting and prolonging it. Ketogenic foods are perfect for this.

The first meal can include the following ingredients:

- Vegetables, such as spinach, broccoli, cauliflower, cabbage, kale, asparagus, artichokes, seaweed, Brussels sprouts, green beans, chard, celery, cucumbers, lettuce or any other type of salad, zucchinis, tomatoes, bell peppers, garlic, onions, squash, mushrooms and blueberries.

- Meat, such as pork chops, chicken thighs/wings, bacon, mince, beef, lamb, venison, liver, heart, kidneys, duck, wild game, such as boar, moose, deer.
- Other sources of protein, such as eggs, salmon, mackerel, herring, sardines, anchovies and sprats.
- Some fats, such as butter, olive oil, tallow, lard, olives, ghee, avocadoes, heavy cream, cheese, nuts and seeds.

Example dishes would include:

- 1-2 strips of bacon with 2-3 eggs and 1 cup of spinach.
- 1 can of sardines with some salad and 1 cup of almonds.
- 1 cup of pork sausage with 1 cup of steamed broccoli covered with butter.

In total, you shouldn't go over 500 calories during the undereating phase.

The idea behind the first meal is to give your body at least some form of nutrients but to still keep it slightly hungry. It's important to get some protein (about 25-40 grams at first), restrict your carb intake (<10 grams) and eat enough healthy fats.

Avoid high amounts of carbohydrates that will spike your insulin and may cause a crash. Don't eat potatoes, rice, grains or fruit, as they'll make you burn sugar instead of fat. Too much sweetness will also create more cravings. You'll also not be satiated by them. Eat some protein, fat and fibrous vegetables as your first meal, so that you'll be satisfied for longer.

When you eat foods high in natural minerals and fiber you're nourishing and satisfying your body, whereas processed food high in carbohydrates leaves you malnourished. This leads to the feeling of deprivation and causes binging. Your brain is simply in an energy crisis and is searching for nutrients. Maximize nutrient density and don't eat empty calories that leave your starving.

The best meals to break a fast that has lasted longer than 24 hours would be something liquid, such as bone broth soup with minerals. You can also have something else that's higher in potassium and alkaline, like an avocado or steamed vegetables. Having heavier food right away isn't ideal because it's harder to digest. Oils and butter are fine, but wait a bit before you eat meat.

At dinner you will be transitioning over from undereating to overfeeding. This is the point where you'll stop fasting and start feasting. Unless you follow a ketogenic diet, you can now eat carbohydrates and not worry about insulin. However, I would still stick to Paleo foods for better health.

The biggest meal can include: the same foods - vegetables, meat, eggs, fish, nuts, seeds, oils etc. But also sweet potatoes, rice, quinoa and other types of healthy carbs, such as carrots, turnips, beetroot. Lentils and beans are fine as well, but because of their high lectin content they should be restricted.

Example dishes would be:

- Cooked salmon with roasted vegetables.
- Roasted pork belly with salad.
- Oven baked sweet potatoes with whitefish.

You'll now be simply eating the rest of your calories, whatever that number may be. Dinner can be quite big, which is why you don't have to consume it in one sitting. I like to take my time and spend about 2-3 hours eating. I'm not constantly chewing but will simply have several plates over the course of the evening.

This is also the perfect time to be with your family and just relax. It's important to step back from the stressful stimuli you've been creating during the day so that your body could recover properly. The positive effect of hormesis lies in just an adequate dose of catabolism.

Here are some of <u>the most empowering superfoods</u> we should be eating on a daily basis and while fasting. They should be staples, no matter what diet you choose to follow. If you want the effects of IF to give you long term health benefits, then you need to couple it with optimal nutrition.

- **Eggs** are the #1 source of natural protein in the world. Their high in omega-3 fatty acids, cholesterol, saturated fat, DHA and EPA, which are all essential for healthy nerve cell and neurotransmitter functioning. They also cover the entire amino acid spectrum and are delicious. The yolk is where all of the vitamins and minerals are hidden, so don't throw them away.

- **Kelp** is a sea vegetable rich in iodine, iron and iron. It promotes healthy thyroid functioning and keeps your hormones in check. These nutrients are hard to come by in other foods. Sea vegetables have high amounts of bioavailable iron and vanadium, the latter of which decreases our body's production of glucose and help us increase our ability to store starch in the form of glucose.

- **Broccoli** has a ton of fiber that's good for colon health and is probably one of the best foods for fighting cancer and tumors. It reduces blood pressure, has anti-aging compounds and improves our immune system. By eating broccoli every single day, you are doing your health a huge favor.

- **Spinach.** Yet another anti-inflammatory and cancer fighting vegetable that tastes amazing. It's also rich in potassium which is important for electrolyte balance and overcoming magnesium deficiencies. The antioxidant benefits will also keep our body clean and provide us with more than enough vitamins. One cup of spinach has 3 times the amount of potassium than one medium sized banana. Also, Popeye eats it as well, and he's quite strong, don't you think?

- **Butter.** It is the most easily absorbable source of vitamin-A, which is necessary for thyroid and adrenal health. It also contains lauric acid, which treats fundal infections and candida. The antioxidants protect against cell free radical damage and the lecithins are essential for cholesterol metabolism. Moreover, is rich in vitamin D, E, K and has many other benefits. Do not confuse it with its hydrogenated bastard brother margarine, which is actually a vegetable oil and highly inflammatory. Those processed trans-fats are literally lethal, as they cause cellular death. Avoid them like wildfire.

- **Coconut oil**. One of the healthies sources of fat in the world. It contains fatty acids with powerful medicinal properties and is made up of 90% saturated fat. Because coconut oil contains mostly medium-chain triglycerides, opposed to the long-chain ones, it gets metabolized faster and more efficiently. This provides immediate energy to the brain and circumvents the slow absorption of fat molecules.

- **Wild-caught oily fish**. Salmon, sardines, trout, sprats, anchovies are all great sources of protein but also full of essential fatty acids, such as omega-3s, DHA and EPA. Eating seafood is great for our brain and will allow our cognition to flourish as well.

- **Organ meats**, such as heart, liver, kidneys and gizzards are where all of the vitamins and minerals are at. In nature, predators would also go for the organs first, to get all of their essential nutrients in. Organ meat isn't actually any different from flesh. They are just denser in nutrients, such as B vitamins, iron, phosphorus, copper and magnesium.

- **Avocados.** Loaded with heart-healthy monounsaturated fatty acids they also contain more potassium than bananas. Eating avocados lowers cholesterol, triglyceride levels and protects against cancer. It can also help you absorb nutrients from other plant foods. One of the biggest benefits of the avocado is that it has one of the highest quantities of pantothenic acid in the world._It's a complex B vitamin and is one of the most important ones. If you're deficient in it, then you won't be able to use your macronutrients as energy as efficiently. Your hormones and immune system would stop working.

These are just a few of the most powerful superfoods in the world. I hope you saw a re-emerging pattern here – most of them are seafood or full of healthy fats. That's right, fat is good for us, unlike we've been led to believe. A lot of modern day doctors also don't advocate fasting and look where we have ended up now.

Here's a list of bullet points to follow for a 24-hour fast:

- Eat dinner the previous night at about 7-8 PM.
- Fast throughout the night and wake up in the morning.
- Drink a big glass of water with some salt in it once you wake up.
- Have some tea and more water the first few hours.
- Wait 2-3 hours before you drink coffee, or longer if you don't get hungry.

- Fast past noon for about 14-16 hours, or go for the 24-hour mark.
- Go for a walk on an empty stomach.
- Before you break your fast, have a glass of hot water with lemon juice squeezed in it.
- Make your first meal relatively small and low-glycemic. Don't exceed 500 calories and don't eat carbohydrates.
- Wait 2-3 hours before you workout at 4PM, or have another meal.
- Workout between 3-6PM.
- Transition over from undereating to overfeeding at 6-7PM.
- Have dinner at 7-8PM.
- Stick to Paleo-esque ketogenic meals for maximum nutrient density.
- Eat as much as you like according to your caloric needs and goals.
- Don't gorge yourself until indulgence.
- Spend time with your family and relax.

Here's the 2 day fast formula for 48-hours:

- Have dinner the previous night before at about 6-8 PM.
- Wake up the next morning and drink water with a pinch of sea salt. You want to stay extra hydrated while fasting.
- When you get hungry don't drink coffee right away and stick to some green tea.
- Wait a few hours until noon and then have a cup of black coffee with nothing added, or continue with drinking tea. Don't drink more than 2-4 cups.
- Another great appetite suppressant is sparkling mineral water.
- Walking, reading, keeping your mind busy and not thinking about fasting will all make the experience very easy. If you think about the fact that you haven't eaten, then you'll surely get hungry. Don't surround yourself with food either, if you're having trouble with cravings.
- Continue drinking water throughout the day until the evening.
- For "*dinner*" you can have some more herbal teas or decaf coffee.
- Feel how your body starts to rev up its metabolism and release growth hormone.
- Go to bed without feeling any hunger. If you drink enough water, then you shouldn't be hungry at all.
- Wake up the next day and repeat the process until you're starting to reach the end.

Before you break your fast it's recommended to reflect on the experience. Come to the realization that it's nothing bad. A 2 day fast is nothing in comparison to a week or a month.

You can definitely adjust this to your preference and the situations you're in. Don't feel obligated to follow a strict routine because you also want to bring in some variation into your daily practice. This will keep your body guessing and *antifragile.*

Chapter XII

Common Mistakes of the Inexperienced Practitioner

Intermittent fasting is incredibly easy – you don't eat and simply drink water. However, there are still some mistakes we can possibly make. This short section of the book will cover the deadly sins and how to avoid making them.

Don't get addicted to coffee.

Caffeine is an incredible appetite suppressant and reduces any hunger for many hours by increasing our focus and giving us energy. At the same time, it can also turn into a powerful drug.

A lot of people are like zombies when it comes to drinking coffee. They wake up, barely crawl out of bed and immediately reach out for a cup. What's worse, they add sugar and milk to it, making it even more stimulating. After the effects of wakefulness have diminished, they make another one and another one until they've become completely numb to it. It's a sad thing to see someone being addicted to anything, even something so seemingly innocent.

As in the case with insulin, the more we release it, the more resistant we become. You get used to running on caffeine and the added dose of sugar can make you feel like you can keep going. To maintain our sensitivity, we have to receive its stimulus less often. While fasting we shouldn't drink more than 2-5 cups of coffee a day, nor should we feel the need to. When in mild ketosis, we'll already be having more energy and caffeine is just a nice thing to have.

I love coffee but I'm always mindful of how much and how often I'm consuming it. It's actually extremely good for us. If the beans are organic and free from mold, then the drink acts like an antioxidant. It also increases fat oxidation and sharpens our cognition. The famous philosopher of the Enlightenment Voltaire used to drink more than 10 cups a day, but I wouldn't recommend you to do that.

One of the best ways to maintain your sensitivity to caffeine is to cycle between regular coffee and decaf. They both taste the same and will suppress your appetite as much. To be honest, there isn't much difference in flavor. I tend to drink decaf for the majority of the week and use regular coffee whenever I feel like I need an extra boost. I'm not dependent of any stimulation and will thus remain *antifragile*.

Don't get dehydrated.

We should instead increase our water intake. Drinking 8 cups of water a day isn't enough, especially while we're fasting. Coffee is a diuretic and will increase dehydration. Compensate that with adding a bit of sea salt into your water. This will improve fluid absorption and keeps the electrolytes in balance. You have to stay hydrated throughout the day. Gulping down 2 liters at once will only make you urinate it all out.

Fast just enough.

At this point I would also like to return to *The Hunger Artist*. In the story, the man was put into a cage at the circus. He breaks his personal record of 40 days but no one is there to recognize it, because the staff forgot to change the sign on which his daily total was displayed. The hunger artist then wastes away, unnoticed and unappreciated.

Many days pass, until the overseer discovers the man buried in the straw nearly dead. He speaks his last words, asking to be forgiven, explaining that he wanted to be admired by everyone. When the overseer tells him that everyone does admire him, the hunger artist says that they shouldn't, confessing that he fasted only because in life he couldn't find food that he liked. Then he died.

The first rule of Fight Club is: you do not talk about the Fight Club.

Don't do fasting to become some sort of a martyr. The 19th century German philosopher Friedrich Nietzsche would agree with me on this: *"Wherever on earth the religious neurosis has appeared we find it tied to three dangerous dietary demands: solitude, fasting, and sexual abstinence. (Beyond Good and Evil : §47)"* Fasting shouldn't be some sort of a means to *"repent our sins."* It's an empowering strategy that causes advantageous metabolic adaptations and hormonal responses, which we use to augment our body.

The second rule of Fight Club is: you do not talk about the Fight Club!

It's not a means of punishing oneself either. We shouldn't do intermittent fasting as restriction but instead as something that liberates and empowers us. Simply doing it in some shape or form is enough.

The third rule of Fight Club is: if someone yells "stop!", goes limp, or taps out, the fight is over.

Self-mastery is also a double-edged sword. It asserts dominance over our unconscious urges but at the same time can be taken too far.

You need to be mindful the conditions of your body and how well you can handle fasting. The fact is that physiologically you'll be fine. It's just that psychologically you may not be prepared for abstaining from food for long periods of time.

Don't jump into it right away if you can't handle it. Start with having 14 hour fasts, then 16, then 18 and then have your first 24-hour fast. If you want to go beyond that, then be my guest, but do so at your own risk and concern.

Fourth rule: only two guys to a fight.

Don't try to impress someone else or get attached to an expected outcome. Fasting is a way to get more in tune with your own body and empower your body. It's you versus yourself, first and foremost.

Bringing in too many other stressors.

Fasting is a hormetic stressor to the body that needs to be taken in the right dose for it to have a positive response. The benefits will kick in only when the stimulus is just enough to force us to adapt but not too much for us to handle. There's a fine line between anxiety and boredom. It's a balancing act that requires a lot of attention and self-awareness.

If you're doing daily fasts of 20+ hours, then you should be mindful of other stressors you may come across. Most common is probably training. It's a lot stronger stimulus than fasting and when you add these two on top of each other you get a very powerful catabolic effect. In the right amounts it can be beneficial, however, in that case you would have to scale down either the intensity or frequency of your exercise. Doing this every single day without giving your body time to recover will over-stimulate your adrenals and lead to adrenal fatigue. That's when you've completely reached burnout and your organism is fighting for its life.

Additional stressors include lack of sleep and excessive exposure to artificial light at night. Blue light in the evening can offset our circadian rhythm and thus block the expression of some hormones. Remember, most of the growth hormone gets released during the first few hours of sleep, at about 11-12PM. If you're on your gadgets at that time, then you may miss out on a lot. At least you won't be able to get into a deep state of repair by that time, as blue light will also stop the production of melatonin, the sleep hormone.

Sleep deprivation lowers testosterone and can cause insulin resistance. Only a few hours of sleep for several nights in a row will make your blood sugar levels rise to that of a diabetic. If you stay there for too long, you'll eventually get sick yourself. Don't think that you can get away with this, because eventually it will catch up with you.

Your body will only start to repair itself when its sleeping. All of the repair mechanisms and waste removal happens at night. That's also when we're building muscle and getting stronger. An adequate stimulus needs to be recovered from for full adaptation to occur.

One last mistake would be to get too cold. It's a stress response like any other, as the body will always try to maintain its core temperature. Shivering is a way to produce endogenous heat and shows that your internal thermostat is working hard. During fasting you may feel more cold than you normally would. If your fingers and toes are getting numb or blue, then you should stop and cover yourself up. Dress warmly and don't push yourself too hard.

Ignoring the signs and soldiering through.

The positive effects of hormesis occur with just the right dosage. If you take it too far then you'll be actually causing more harm than good. Adaptations occur gradually and need to happen progressively. At first your body won't be able to cope with fasting as well as it will later. Your fat burning ketogenic pathways have to be re-created before you can effectively utilize them.

Some signs of too much fasting are constant headaches, fatigue, feeling like being hit with a club, not sleeping well, shivering and feeling very cold despite wearing a lot of clothes. Be mindful of how your body reacts and listen to the signs that you're being given. Pushing it too far will lead to burnout and won't result with an advantageous outcome.

Gorging after fasting.

Intermittent fasting loses all of its beauty if you still eat like a scavenger all the time. It shouldn't be a means of eating more food, but a way to get away with eating less, without losing muscle and strength.

The Buddha also realized this, as he found that complete abstinence wasn't necessary. After he broke his 72 day fast, he started practicing moderation instead. That's the key idea we should take away here. When it comes to eating, walk the golden path in the middle. But also practice antifragility, which is by nature an extreme event.

Don't eat whatever.

Intermittent fasting is a great way to create a caloric deficit. Because you'll be eating less often, your meals can be larger in quantities and calories. This can also mean that you're able to eat some junk food, while still maintaining a negative energy balance.

For *if it fits your macros* (IIFYM) type of flexible dieting it may work, but it's not optimal for overall health. Of course, the 80-20 rule can be applied here as well, and some indulgence here and there does you no harm.

At the same time, you should also consider what you're trying to accomplish with your nutrition in general. Is food just calories, or is it something more powerful? One thing is certain – eating causes certain metabolic adaptations and processes within the body. The hormonal response is a lot more important for longevity.

That's why I'm following a ketogenic diet. It's a low carb approach that restricts carbohydrate intake to less than 30-50 grams per day. This puts the body into a state of nutritional ketosis, which happens after prolonged fasting as well. After a while, a complete shift in metabolism takes place and you'll be utilizing ketones as your primary fuel source, instead of glucose.

The keto diet mimics the physiology of fasting but has other additional metabolic advantages. It will skyrocket your energy levels and increases mitochondrial density (the nuclear power plants of our cells). The benefits of fasting primarily have to do with ketone and fat utilization at the expense of glucose depletion. Ketosis puts us into a higher gear of fat burning, which influences not only fat oxidation, but also the entire body.

If you're interested about learning more about this miraculous, yet mysterious, condition, then make sure you check out my other books in the Simple Keto series.

Chapter XIII

Supplementation

Despite our access to abundant contemporary food we're still missing some key ingredients - the micronutrients. To overcome this flaw there are some supplements we should be taking.

With the industrialization of food all of that has suffered. Our soils are being depleted from their vital life force with the use of fertilizers, spraying of toxic fumes, usage of GMOs, radiation, travel pollution and many other things. All for the purpose of creating more empty calories and food without any actually beneficial content.

A word of caution. There are a lot of supplements we could be taking. However, that doesn't mean we should start gorging on piles of tablets and numerous pills. It's not about becoming a substance junkie, but a self-empowered being who simply covers all of the necessary micronutrients through the usage of natural yet still manufactured additives.

We don't need to take a whole lot, simply some which everyone needs and especially those that we're individually most deficient of. That's something we have to find out ourselves.

We don't need to fear these pharmaceuticals just because their artificial form. They are just natural ingredients that have been processed and put into a bottle or a powder.

All of the supplements that I have listed here are least processed and free from any additional garbage, such as preservatives, GMO, gluten, starch, sugar etc. They're keto-proof and friendly.

Additionally, we should always try to stick to real whole foods as much as possible. Supplements are just that - supplementation for some of the deficiencies we fail to get from what we actually eat. They're not magical but simply give us the extra edge.

The effects these products have can be derived from natural foods as well. In the form of a pill or a powder they're simply microscopic and packaged nutrition. Taking them will grant us access to optimal health - the utmost level of wellbeing and performance both physical and mental.

In this list are all of the supplements I am personally taking because of their importance, as well as the additional benefits we get. However, I do not advise anyone to take any of them unless they are aware of their medical condition and don't know about the possible side effects or issues that may or may not follow.

Before taking anything we ought to educate ourselves about the topic and consult a professional physician. <u>The responsibility is solely on the individual and I will take none.</u>

<u>Natural Seasoning</u>

To start off I'm going to list the supplements we should be taking, each and every one of us, as they are something that we're definitely all deficient of and also promote Superhuman wellbeing.

Not everything we consume ought to come in the form of a pill. A lot of micronutrients can be found in unprocessed products as well, we simply need to add them to our diet and reap the benefits. They are most natural and completely free from the touch of man. Therefore, they come first and are of utmost value.

- **Turmeric.** One of the best spices we can use is curcumin or turmeric. It has a lot of medicinal properties, such as anti-inflammatory compounds, increase of antioxidants and brain health. Also, it fights and prevents many diseases, such as Arthritis, Alzheimer's and even cancer. In addition to that, it tastes amazing and can be added to everything. I sprinkle it on all foods and run out quite quickly which is why I also buy it in bulk so that it's cheaper. You can also take a capsule.

- **Ginger.** Continuing on with turmeric's brother. It has almost as much health benefits. In addition to that, it lowers blood sugar levels, fights heart disease, treats chronic indigestion, may reduce menstrual pain for women, lowers cholesterol and heals muscle pain. Once again, <u>bulk</u> or <u>capsule</u>.

- **Cinnamon.** These three create the most important natural spices we should be eating on a daily basis. They're incredibly cheap and easy to come by yet have amazing health as well as performance enhancing benefits. Moreover, they all make food taste amazing. Cinnamon falls into the same category as ginger and turmeric - superfoods, because it truly empowers us. In addition to the same medicinal properties it also increases insulin sensitivity, fights neurodegenerative disease and bacterial infections. What's best about it is that it can be added to not only salty foods but on desserts as well. I even add it to my coffee. The best to use is <u>Ceylon</u> or „true" cinnamon.

- **Green tea.** It isn't an actual supplement but is still extremely empowering. In fact, it can be considered to be the healthiest beverage of the world after water. It improves health, brain function, fat oxidation and detoxifies the system. Additionally, lowers blood pressure and prevents all types of disease, including Alzheimer's and cancer. We don't need to take pills with extracts but can get all of the benefits by simply drinking a cup a day. However, to get all of the benefits we need to be consuming about 15-30 cups. Using a capsule would be very efficient.

- **Garlic.** It has a strong taste and smell but is incredibly healthy nonetheless. Chopping garlic cloves forms a compound called allicin, which, once digested, travels all over the body and exerts its potent biological effects. It fights all illness, especially the cold, reduces blood pressure, improves cholesterol levels, contains antioxidants, increases longevity, detoxifies the body from metals, promotes bone health and is delicious. Because of its flavor it makes a great addition to meals. It also comes in capsuled form.

Supplements you HAVE to Take

Moving on with actual supplements. These things we're all deficient of and they also take our performance to the next level, they empower us.

- **Fish/Krill oil.** It's rich in omega-3 fatty acids, which are great for the brain and heart. The counterpart to that is omega-6, which are pro-inflammatory and bad for us. Omega-6 can be found in a lot of processed foods and vegetable oils, which we would want to avoid anyway. For our body to be healthy the omega-3's need to be in balance with the omega-6's. Unfortunately, that balance can be easily tipped off as every amount of omega-6 requires triple the amount of omega-3 to reduce the negative effects. Additionally, fish oil has DHA, which promotes brain functioning, fights inflammation, supports bone health, increases physical performance etc. Naturally, it can be found in fatty fish such as salmon, herring, mackerel and sardines. Fish oil falls into the same category because of its vital importance for superhuman health. It can be used easily as a capsule or liquidized.

Taking one teaspoon a day will drastically improve your life. Krill oil might simply be a more potent and bioavailable source. Make sure to use wild caught sources to avoid mercury poisoning.

- **Vitamin D-3.** This is the sunshine vitamin and is one of the most important nutrients. Life exists on Earth because of the Sun. D-3 governs almost every function within us starting from DNA repair and metabolic processes making it a foundation to everything that goes on. It's embedded in nutritious food, given it has received enough exposure to solar light. Vitamin D-3 fights cardiovascular, autoimmune and infective diseases. Of course, the best source would be to get it from the Sun but that is not always possible because of seasonality and location. It can be consumed as oil or a capsule.

- **Magnesium.** Another foundational mineral. It comprises 99% of the body's mineral content and governs almost all of the processes. Magnesium helps to build bones, enables nerves to function and is essential for the production of energy from food. This is especially beneficial for the physically active. Some people who are depressed get headaches because of this deficiency. Because our soils are quite depleted magnesium needs to be <u>supplemented</u>. It can also be used as an <u>oil</u> on your skin for greater absorption in specific areas.

Supplements Empowered

We have covered all of the supplements we should be taking no matter what, the most important and essential ones. Now I'll get down to the empowering ones.

They are not foundational but beneficial nonetheless. With the help of these we can transcend the boundary between healthy and superhuman performance as they will take us to the next level.

- **Creatine Monohydrate.** Creatine is an organic acid produced in the liver that helps to supply energy to cells all over the body, especially muscles. It enhances ATP production and allows for muscle fibers to contract faster, quicker, and makes them overall stronger. That means increased physical performance with explosive and strength based movements and sprinting. However, it doesn't end there. Creatine has been found to improve cognitive functioning, as it's a nootropic as well, improving mental acuity and memory. Naturally, it can be found most in red meat. It's <u>dirty cheap</u> and easy to consume, as only 5 grams per day will do wonders and doing so won't make a person big nor bulky.

- **Pro- and prebiotics.** Having a well working digestive system is incredibly vital for getting the most nutrients out of our food. Industrialization has done another disservice to us by destroying all of the bacteria in the food we consume, the good and the bad, and replacing them with preservatives. We might be eating but we're not actually deriving a lot of nutrients. In order to have a healthy gut we need to have a well-functioning microbiome. Naturally, food is full of living organisms. Sauerkraut, raw milk, yoghurt, unprocessed meat all have good bacteria in them. With there being no life in our food, we need to create it within us ourselves. <u>Probiotics</u> are alive microorganisms in a pill that transport these good

195

bacteria into our gut for improved digestion and immune system. <u>Prebiotics</u> are different, they're not alive, but plant fiber that feeds the bacteria. They're indigestible parts of the vegetable that go through our digestive track into our gut where the bacteria then eat them. If you don't like eating a lot of broccoli and spinach, then you should still get a lot of fiber into your diet.

- **Thyroid supplementation.** The thyroid gland is incredibly important for our health because it regulates the functioning of our metabolism. Moreover, because of its location in our throat it also is a connective point between the brain and the rest of the body. This organ is a part of an incredibly complex system which creates this intertwined relationship between the two. With a low functioning thyroid one will have an impeded metabolism, suffer hypothyroidism and many other diseases because of the necessary hormones will not be produced. Promoting thyroid functioning can be done by taking <u>iodine supplementation</u> or eating a lot of <u>sea vegetables</u>. The daily requirements for selenium can be met with eating only 2-3<u>Brazil nuts</u>.

- **Multivitamin.** There are definitely a lot of vitamins to be covered for our body to not only be healthy but function at its peak. It would be unreasonable to take too many tablets or pills while neglecting the importance of real food. However, taking a multivitamin that has a lot of beneficial minerals all combined into one bottle is very effective and will most definitely be useful.

- **Maca.** Another superfood comes from the Peruvian mountains and is the root of ginseng. It has numerous amounts of vitamins and minerals in it, such as magnesium zinc, copper etc. Also, it promotes hormone functioning for both men and women, as well as increases our energy production just like creatine does. It can either be powdered or made into a tablet.

- **GABA.** Called gamma-aminobutyric acid, it's the main inhibitory neurotransmitter, and regulates the nerve impulses in the human body. Therefore, it is important for both physical and mental performance, as both of them are connected to the nervous system. Also, GABA is to an extent responsible for causing relaxation and calmness, helping to produce BDNF.

- **Chaga mushroom.** Chaga is a mushroom that grows on birch trees. It's extremely beneficial for supporting the immune system, has anti-oxidative and soothing properties, lowers blood pressure and cholesterol. Also, consuming it will promote the health and integrity of the adrenal glands. This powder can be added to teas or other warm beverages. Or you can grind it yourself.

- **MCT oil.** For nutritional ketosis having an additional source of ketone bodies will be beneficial. MCT stands for medium chain triglycerides which are fat molecules that can be digested more rapidly than normal fat ones, which are usually long chain triglycerides. Doing so will enable the brain to have immediate access to abundant energy and a deeper state of ketosis. Basically, it's glucose riding the vessel of ketones. Naturally, it's extracted from coconut oil and is an enhanced liquidized version of it. Additionally, I also eat raw coconut flakes, which have MCTs in them.

- **Collagen protein.** Collagen provides the fastest possible healthy tissue repair, bone renewal and recovery after exercise. It can also boost mental clarity, reduce inflammation, clear your skin, promote joint integrity, reduces aging and builds muscle. Naturally, it's found in tendons and ligaments, that can be consumed by eating meat. As a supplement it can be used as <u>protein powder</u> or as <u>gelatin capsules</u>.

- **Branched Chain Amino Acids.** L-Leucine, L-Isoleucine, and L-Valine are grouped together and called BCAAs because of their unique chemical structure. They're essential and have to be derived from diet. Supplementing them will increase performance, muscle recovery and protein synthesis. There is no solid evidence to show any significant benefit to BCAAs. However, they can be very useful <u>to take</u> before fasted workouts to reduce muscle catabolism.

This was just a small bonus chapter for you to improve the quality of your nutrition. Intermittent fasting is great but we should also be mindful about getting enough micronutrients into our feasts.

Bonus Chapter

Get in Touch with Your Primal Instinct

Throughout this book I've been referring to this mythical primal instinct over and over again. It's an innate part of our physiology and inside all of us.

Even those slaves in Ancient Rome had it. Their beast had simply been domesticated and was lying dormant, waiting to be awoken. Spartacus was able to ignite courage in their hearts again and break the chains of bondage.

Ever heard about feats of Superhuman strength? A mother lifting up a car to save her child. Or a grandfather leaping up to a tree to escape from stray dogs. That's what I'm talking about. We're capable of a lot more than we think.

By default, we're supposed to not use our Superhuman abilities. Our own mind creates a block so that we could prevent ourselves from too much exertion. Energy in the ancestral savannah was scarce and we will unleash our killer instinct only in situations of life and death.

In the modern world we don't come across enough stimulus that would make us tap into our inner beast. It's our secret weapon that will lose its effect unless we use it. That's why we ought to deliberately condition our body to release this power from time to time.

Intermittent fasting is one of the catalysts that helps us to get in touch with our primal instinct. However, it's not enough to let it loose. To break the cage, we also have to face a situation where our body experiences extreme exertion and catabolism. It functions as a point of no return. We either sink or swim.

We don't have to run away from lions or wrestle with bears anymore, but creating these survival scenarios will be very beneficial for our physiology. The hormetic effect will not only make us stronger physically, but will also make us mentally more resistant to stress.

High intensity training, in any shape or form, stimulates the sympathetic nervous system and causes immense stress to the body. It's also very good for our cardiovascular fitness and longevity. On top of that, it increases our mitochondrial density, which are the power plants of our cells.

At those times we'll be gasping for air and fighting for our existence. It's incredibly powerful and will yield extreme anabolic effects.

In comparison to steady state cardio, high intensity interval training is a lot more effective. As with the case of getting stronger – you have to actually lift heavy weights. Your body won't adapt to novel circumstances unless you condition yourself with facing them.

The best type of high intensity training is HIIT cardio and resistance training. I suggest you implement them into your exercise routine and forget about jogging completely. Barbell squats, handstand push-ups, hill sprints, burpees, kettlebell swings – you name it. Whatever your choice might bet. Simply start doing them.

Training fasted adds on top of the hormonal response you'll be creating. It will skyrocket fat oxidation and HGH release.

Once you reach your 90% maximum and stay in that zone for some time, you'll be incredibly catabolic. In response, your body will react by releasing more adrenalin into your blood stream and will also unleash your killer instinct. As far as your subconscious mind can tell, you're fighting for your life.

During fasted high intensity training you'll experience a different type of focus and determination. Your movements will be precise and there will be nothing else on your mind other than the task at hand. It's a unique sensation and definitely empowering.

Here's a sample HIIT routine.

My favourite type of HIIT cardio are either burpees or sprinting. It's easy and you can max out on them completely without sacrificing good form.

- 30 seconds of burpees/sprinting

- Rest for 30 seconds to a minute.
- Repeat for about 5-10 rounds.

In total, this workout shouldn't take you longer than 15 minutes and is a lot more time-efficient than steady state cardio. To create some real adaptations in your physiology, you have to give it some serious reasons for doing so. Training should be more than simply a way to burn calories.

Paradoxically, some of my best training happens when I'm in a fasted or at least underfed state. I've managed to hit some significant personal records despite not having eaten anything for 20+ hours.

It's actually a very strange experience, almost enlightening, if you will. Your body is under intense physical conditions, your heart is pounding like crazy, you can feel the adrenaline and cortisol pumping through your veins – it's chaos. Yet, there's pure stillness, consciousness and total self-mastery. You'll feel like standing at the door step of infinite potentiality.

At those times I find myself asking: *"How much further can I go?"* Then, only my own limitations can keep me down and impossible literally becomes a word.

Keep in mind that this is an extreme stress response. You won't experience growth unless you supercompensate for it. Repair mechanisms will kick in during overfeeding, sleeping and take some time. Self-mastery is a double-edged sword and can cause some severe battle wounds, if pushed too far.

High intensity training in conjunction with fasting hits our body with a hammer and unleashes our inner beast. Use this weapon wisely, but don't over-do it.

Conclusion

Becoming a Fat Burning Beast

Can you feel it? Can you feel your growth hormone and testosterone levels rising? Well I certainly do, because I'm fasting at the moment. Once you start practicing the pattern of undereating and overfeeding you'll be able to feel the same way.

What's more, you'll improve your health, performance and longevity. The resistance to stress and mental toughness that you cultivate will transition over to every other area of your life as well. You simply have to teach your body to adapt.

Intermittent fasting is a way to make ourselves better at using fat for fuel. The notion here isn't about burning calories, but in the way your body is utilizing its energy sources.

But it doesn't end there. In order to become a fat burning beast we have to do a lot more. That's why I support the ketogenic diet. It's an altered metabolic state in which you've completely shifted from using glucose to solely ketones. This makes us even more in tune with our primal instinct.

I advise you to try out the keto diet, at least once. This is important for your body to experience what it feels like to burn fat and create these aboriginal ketogenic pathways within you. Intermittent fasting isn't enough. You have to restrict your carbohydrate intake to a bare minimum.

Luckily, I've written a series of books about the ketogenic diet for various circumstances. They're listed at the end. Check them out.

I'm also going to share with you a concept of mine called optimal nutrition. It can be grasped under a single sentence, which goes as follows:

Optimal nutrition is eating the right things, in the right amounts at the right time.

I do not know about you but I think there cannot be made a better definition than that. It covers all of what we need to know OBJECTIVELY, meaning that it is not taken out of context and can be applied to any situation. We simply need to decipher it and make it fit our demands.

Intermittent fasting is a huge part of that, but it may not fit into the paradigm of optimal nutrition all of the time. For the most part it does. Even myself who trains quite hard feels this way.

On this note I'm going to end the book.

Stay Empowered

Siim

More Books from the Author

Read more books in my Simple Keto series.

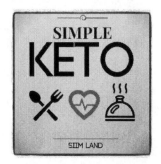

Simple Keto the Easiest Ketogenic Diet Book

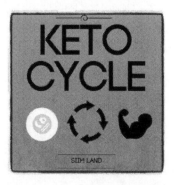

Keto Cycle the Cyclical Ketogenic Diet Book

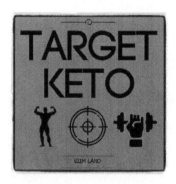

Target Keto the Targeted Ketogenic Diet Book

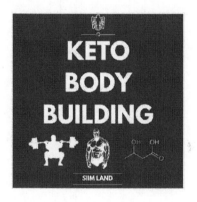

Keto Bodybuilding: Build Lean Muscle and Burn Fat at the Same Time by Eating a Low Carb Ketogenic Bodybuilding Diet and Get the Physique of a Greek God

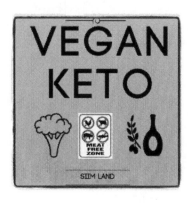

Vegan Keto: the Vegan Ketogenic Diet

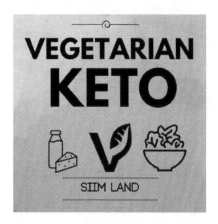

Vegetarian Keto: Start a Plant Based Low Carb High Fat Vegetarian Ketogenic Diet to Burn Fat and Improve Insulin Sensitivity

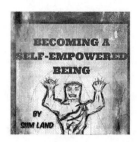

Becoming a Self Empowered Being

Leave a Review on Amazon!

If you liked this book, then I would appreciate it, if you could leave a 5-star review on Amazon. It helps me out a ton and is the least you can do to help other people start a ketogenic diet as well.

About the Author

My name is Siim Land. In addition to writing books such as this I run a blog at http://siimland.com. I'm also the hero of my own journey. A thinker, writer and a self-empowered being. Pursuing mastery over myself and my craft. Working on achieving my truest potential. After finishing high school I went through 8 months of military service during which I learned to control my own thoughts and actions. The competence on the topic of self-mastery is the result of that period as well as the constant process of self-actualization that occurred later in my life. Also an undergraduate in anthropology I intend to continue this path of development. My approach is holistic by nature taking into account every aspect of our lives. This way no stone will be left unturned and the best results achieved. This includes the body-mind-soul triumvirate. For future updates about my personal growth and more useful information for you head over to my website.

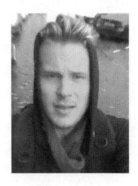

Contact me at my blog: http://www.siimland.com/contact/

References

---

i Oswalt, W H. (1976). *An Anthropological Analysis of Foodgetting Technology.* New York, NY: Wiley.

ii http://www.ncbi.nlm.nih.gov/pubmed/26013791

iii MacSwiney dies after fasting 74 days; npws excites Ireland; riot in Belfast; second hunger striker is dead in Cork; Joseph Murphy dies of 76 days' hunger strike, the second prisoner to succumb in Cork jail. New York Times 1920 Nov 26; 70:1

iv Downie L: Prisoners end fasting in Belfast. The Washington Post 1981 Oct 4, p 1

v Dr. Tanner's fast. Br Med J 1880 Jul 31; 2:171

vi Paton DN, Stockman R: Observations on the metabolism of man during starvation. Proc R Acad Edinb 1888-1889; pp 121-131

vii Rcbins GN: The fasting man. Br Med J 1890 Jun 21; 1: 1444-1446 9. Benedict FG: A Study of Prolonged Fasting, Publication No. 203. Washington DC, Carnegie Institute, 1915

viii Thomson TJ, Runcie J, Miller V: Treatment of obesity by total fasting for up to 249 days. Lancet 1966 Nov 5; 2:992-996

ix Stewart WK, Fleming LW: Features cf a successful therapeutic fast of 382 days' duration. Postgrad Med J 1973 Mar; 49: 203-209

x http://www.ncbi.nlm.nih.gov/pubmed/21847109

xi Owen OE, Felig P, Morgan AP, et al: Liver and kidney metabolism during prolonged starvation. J Clin Invest 1969 Mar; 48:574-583

xii http://www.ncbi.nlm.nih.gov/pubmed/6409904

xiii http://www.ncbi.nlm.nih.gov/pubmed/11757079

xiv http://www.ncbi.nlm.nih.gov/pmc/articles/PMC3583887/

xv http://www.ncbi.nlm.nih.gov/pmc/articles/PMC3106288/

xvi http://www.ncbi.nlm.nih.gov/pubmed/17291990/

xvii http://www.jnutbio.com/article/S0955-2863(04)00261-X/abstract?cc=y=

xviii http://www.ncbi.nlm.nih.gov/pubmed/24048020

[xix] Tunstall RJ, et al. Fasting activates the gene expression of UCP3 independent of genes necessary for lipid transport and oxidation in skeletal muscle. Biochemical and Biophysical Research Communications 2002; 294:301-308

[xx] http://www.ncbi.nlm.nih.gov/pubmed/2405717

[xxi] http://www.ncbi.nlm.nih.gov/pubmed/15640462

[xxii] http://www.ncbi.nlm.nih.gov/pmc/articles/PMC329619/

[xxiii] Merimee TJ, Fineberg SE: Growth hormone secretion in starvation: A reassessment. J Clin Endocrinol Metab 1974 Aug; 39:385-386

[xxiv] Palmblad J, Levi L, Burger A, et al: Effects of total energy withdrawal (fasting) on the levels of growth hormone, thyrotropin, cortisol, adrenaline, noradrenaline, T4, T3, and rT3 in healthy males. Acta Med Scand 1977; 201:15-22

[xxv] Roth J, Glick SM, Yalow RS, et al: Secretion of human growth hormone: Physiologic and experimental modification. Metabolism 1963 Jul; 12:577-579

Beck P, Koumans JT, Winterling CA, et al: Studies of insulin and growth hormone secretion in human obesity. J Lab Clin Med 1964 Oct; 64:654-667

[xxvi] http://www.ncbi.nlm.nih.gov/pubmed/8156941/

[xxvii] http://online.liebertpub.com/doi/10.1089/rej.2014.1624

[xxviii] http://jn.nutrition.org/content/31/3/363.full.pdf

[xxix] http://www.ncbi.nlm.nih.gov/pubmed/11220789

[xxx] http://www.ncbi.nlm.nih.gov/pubmed/17881524/

[xxxi] http://www.ncbi.nlm.nih.gov/pubmed/22548651/

[xxxii] http://www.ncbi.nlm.nih.gov/pmc/articles/PMC2622429/

[xxxiii] Bloom WL: Fasting as an introduction to the treatment of obesity. Metabolism 1959 May; 8:214-220

[xxxiv] http://www.jstor.org/stable/2743982?seq=1#page_scan_tab_contents

[xxxv] http://www.ncbi.nlm.nih.gov/pubmed/19945408

[xxxvi] http://www.cell.com/cell-metabolism/abstract/S1550-4131(13)00454-3

[xxxvii] http://www.cell.com/cell/abstract/S0092-8674(07)01685-6?_returnURL=http%3A%2F%2Flinkinghub.elsevier.com%2Fretrieve%2Fpii%2FS0092867407016856%3Fshowall%3Dtrue&cc=y=

[xxxviii] Williams RH (Ed): Textbook of Endocrinology-5th Ed. Philadelphia, WB Saunders, 1974

[xxxix] http://www.ncbi.nlm.nih.gov/pubmed/23456944?dopt=Abstract

[xl] Grimm O. Addicted to food. Scientific American Mind 2007; 18(2):36-39

[xli] Ganley, R M. 1989. "Emotion and Eating in Obesity: A Review of the Literature." International Journal of Eating Disorders 8 (3): 343–361.

[xlii] Bloom WL: Inhibition of salt excretion by carbohydrate. Arch Intern Med 1962 Jan; 109:80-86 48.

Veverbrants E, Arky RA: Effects of fasting and refeedingI. Studies on sodium, potassiulm and water excretion on a constant electrolyte and fluid intake. J Clin Endocrinol 1969 Jan; 29:55-62 49.

Botulter PR, Hoffman RS, Arky RA: Pattern of sodiuLm excretion accompanying starvation. Metabolism 1973 May; 22: 675-683

[xliii] Chandra R, Liddle RA Cholecystokinin . Curr Opin Endocrinol Diabetes Obes. (2007)

Storr M, et al Endogenous CCK depresses contractile activity within the ascending myenteric reflex pathway of rat ileum . Neuropharmacology. (2003)

[xliv] Geraedts MC, et al Direct induction of CCK and GLP-1 release from murine endocrine cells by intact dietary proteins . Mol Nutr Food Res. (2011)

[xlv] Soeters MR, et al Intermittent fasting does not affect whole-body glucose, lipid, or protein metabolism . Am J Clin Nutr. (2009)

Stote KS, et al A controlled trial of reduced meal frequency without caloric restriction in healthy, normal-weight, middle-aged adults . Am J Clin Nutr. (2007)

[xlvi] http://examine.com/faq/is-it-better-to-do-aerobic-exercise-fasted/

[xlvii] http://link.springer.com/article/10.1007%2Fs00421-009-1289-x

[xlviii] Knapik JJ, Jones BH, Meredith C, Evans WJ. Influence of a 3.5 day fast on physical performance. European Journal of Applied Physiology and Occupational Physiology 1987; 56(4):428-32

[xlix] Deuel HJ Jr, Gulick M: Studies on ketosis-I. The sexual variation in starvation ketosis. J Biol Chem 1932 Apr; 96:25-34

[l] Bloom WL, Azar G, Clark J, et al: Comparison of metabolic changes in fasting obese and lean patients. Ann NY Acad Sci 1965 Oct 8; 131:623-631

Bloom WL, Azar G, Clark JE: Electrolyte and lipid metabolism of lean fasting men and women. Metabolism 1966 May; 15: 401-408

[li] Merimee TJ, Misbin RI, Pulkkinen AJ: Sex variations in free fatty acids and ketones during fasting: Evidence for a role of glucagon. J Clin Endocrinol Metab 1978 Mar; 46:414-419

[lii] Merimee TJ, Fineberg SE: Homeostasis during fasting-II. Hormone substrate differences between men and women. J Clin Endocrinol Metab 1973 Nov; 37:698-702

Made in the USA
Monee, IL
26 July 2020

37034730R00122